the perfect body
the pilates way

The complete plan for
top to toe transformation

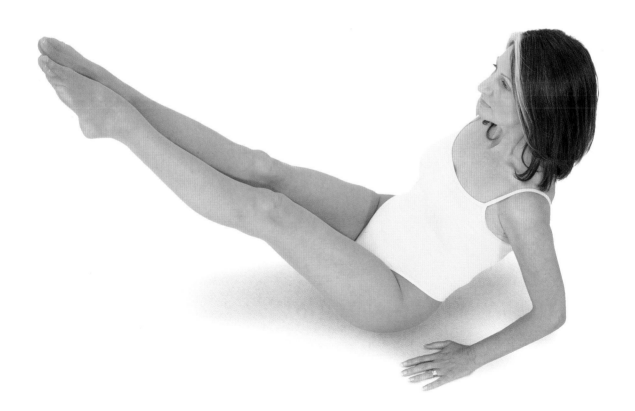

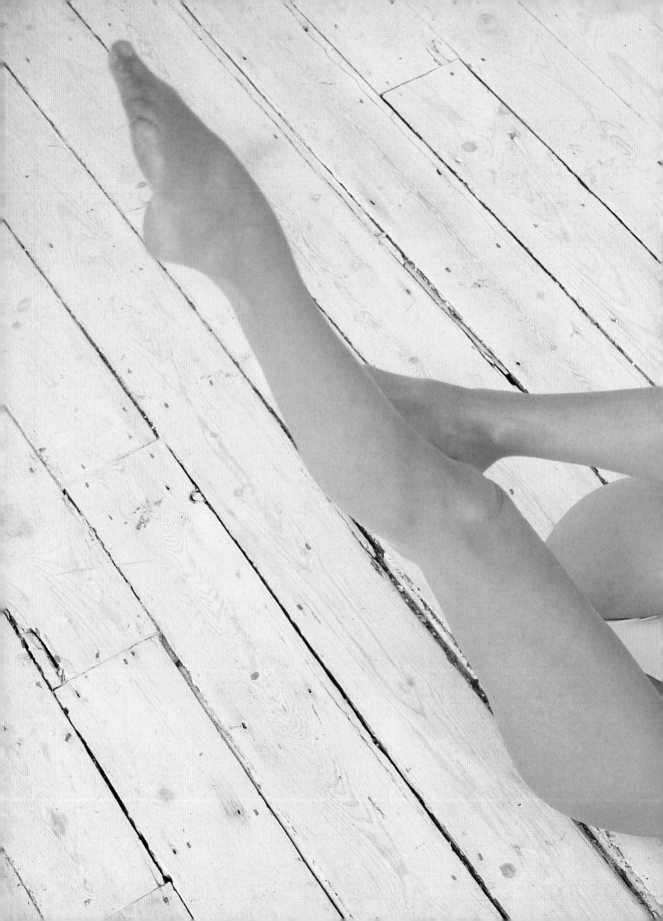

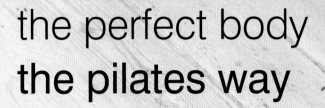

the perfect body
the pilates way

The complete plan for
top to toe transformation

Lynne Robinson
& Caroline Brien

photography by Jim Marks

Macmillan

First published 2002 by Macmillan
an imprint of Pan Macmillan Ltd
Pan Macmillan, 20 New Wharf Road, London N1 9RR
Basingstoke and Oxford
Associated companies throughout the world
www.panmacmillan.com

ISBN 0 333 90752 3

Photography by Jim Marks unless otherwise stated
Food photography by Philip Wilkins
Home economist Mandy Phipps
Recipes by Fiona Hunter
Illustrations by Thorbjorn Ingason

9 8 7 6 5 4 3 2 1

A CIP catalogue record for this book
is available from the British Library.

Typeset by SX Composing DTP, Rayleigh, Essex
Printed and bound in Great Britain
by Butler and Tanner, Frome Somerset

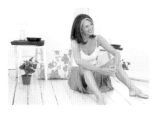

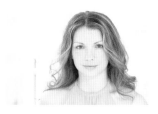

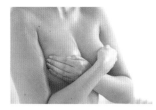

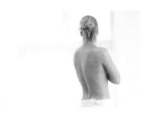

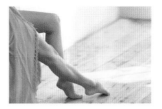

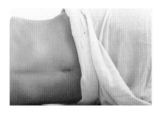

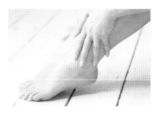

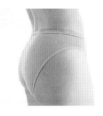

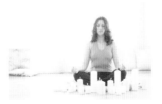

Contents

Acknowledgements

Not in my wildest dreams could I ever have imagined that I would one day write a book entitled 'The Perfect Body'! For most of my life my body was sorely neglected, years of appalling posture, the wrong diet, two heavy babies, a virtual lack of any form of exercise – I think you can begin to imagine what I looked like. But what I also remember was how I felt – simply awful. Plagued with guilt because I was too lazy to follow a healthy lifestyle, I also felt terrible because my body wasn't functioning well. I suffered a variety of ailments ranging from digestive problems to back problems, headaches and eczema.

It is very easy to criticize beauty books and magazines for being superficial and trivial, but most contain sound advice on skincare, diet and exercise. No one is going to claim that using a new salt scrub is going to make you happy or that doing six Spine Curls a day will solve all your problems. But, by making a few simple changes to your daily routine, taking the time to exercise properly, to relax, to shop for a balanced diet, even following a basic skin-care regime, you can both feel and look better, and achieve optimum health. For me, the change to a healthier way of living gave me control again over my body – my body is fitter now at forty-eight than it was at twenty-eight.

I don't know what 'the perfect body' is. I doubt that you could find two people to agree on a definition. It certainly isn't the painfully thin models who often appear in fashion magazines, or the 'surgically enhanced' models that some men's magazines and the tabloids favour. We all have the right to feel good about our bodies, but we should not assume that natural health and beauty comes easily – it requires commitment and discipline. What is clear, however, is that by adopting a healthier lifestyle we give ourselves to chance to realize our true potential.

This is an ideal opportunity for me to thank all the practitioners who have helped me improve my own health, beauty and fitness. I have had the privilege to work with some wonderful Pilates teachers – Gordon Thomson, Miranda Bass and Lisa Bradshaw, in particular, have been a source of inspiration for me. Dr Daya, Fiona Hunter and Raj Jagdev, you have both helped me enormously, enlightening me on diet and overall health. Dene, Gene, Vaishaly – you have kept me looking at my best, thank you all!

And finally, when I need to escape I head for one of two wonderful spas. Twice a year I both relax and work (as a Pilates consultant) at the most luxurious health spa in the world, Chiva Som (Haven of Life) in Thailand. I always return from my trips there rejuvenated and refreshed. My other bolt hole, where we have a Pilates studio, is the Hotel Fortina Spa in Sliema, Malta, where I can combine healthy eating with spa treatments, and of course, Body Control Pilates sessions. As I'm something of a workaholic, these trips have become life savers for me.

Last but by no means least I would like to thank everyone involved in creating this book: Caroline for her enthusiasm, thorough research, patience and endless knowledge; Jim Marks for his sense of humour and understanding of the need for sympathetic lighting; Lisa Valencia for making me look like I should be in the book! And of course the lovely models who so kindly gave up their time, at short notice, to be photographed – Jenny Heanen, Rachel Waldron and Charlotte Thomas.

Lynne Robinson

How To Use This Book

Firstly, I would like to thank Lynne. You know how to make hard work seem like fun and you can always motivate me to do that little bit more. I am also indebted to Fiona Hunter for her excellent nutritional guidance and mouth-watering recipes; as well as the creative Jim Marks, talented Lisa Valencia and gorgeous Victoria Scriven for helping to create such beautiful images. To Gordon Wise, Charlie Mounter and Rafi Romaya at Macmillan, thanks for the opportunity to bring a great idea to life and execute it brilliantly. Thanks, too, to Michael Alcock for your good business sense. To Eve Cameron, Vanessa Raphaely and Catherine Turner, I owe you each a great deal for inspiring and guiding me from the start; and to Susan Harmsworth, Noella Gabriel and Nicky Kinnaird, my deepest gratitude for sharing your insightful knowledge with me both in this book and over the years. Last, but by no means least, special thanks to Justin and my parents Mary and Robert for your love, support and keeping me sane no matter how many deadlines I have!

Caroline Brien

Each chapter of this book focuses on a particular part of the body, tackling common concerns with that area, and combining the latest solutions from the worlds of Pilates, beauty, health and nutrition. As well as explaining how the Body Control Pilates system works (with graded exercises for beginners, intermediate and advanced students), the book also includes simple advice on skincare, aromatherapy, reflexology and massage techniques, giving it a unique approach that fits easily into a modern lifestyle.

Above all, we hope you enjoy using this book. Let it be your body bible and make the most of the time you spend on yourself.

Please note that certain exercises, massage techniques and essential oils are not suitable for use during pregnancy. Please seek advice from your midwife, doctor or qualified practitioner before using those mentioned in this book. Remember, it is always wise for anyone to consult their doctor before taking up a new exercise regime. For example, many of these exercises are wonderful for back-related problems, but you should always seek expert guidance first.

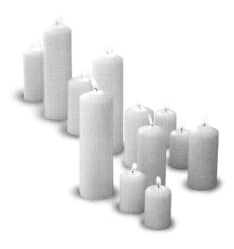

IT'S IRONIC that in an age when we are struggling to achieve perfection in every area of our lives, the amount of time we are able to dedicate to looking good is diminishing. In our world of multi-tasking, life is about instant results and quick-fix solutions, but it takes dedication to reap the benefits of a healthy lifestyle.

The good news, however, is that by adopting a new approach to your body, the results will be long-lasting.

With this in mind, **The Perfect Body the Pilates Way** is a truly holistic and definitive guide to looking good – top to toe, inside and out, mind and body. Improving the way you look is no longer just about what you put on your face or how you spend your time in the gym, it's about how you treat your body as a whole.

Today, the perfect body is one that looks good, works smoothly and is the best you can make it. Your appearance is a reflection of what you eat, what you wear and how you live your life as well as the exercises you do and the beauty regime you follow. Quite simply, it takes a holistic approach to achieve your perfect body.

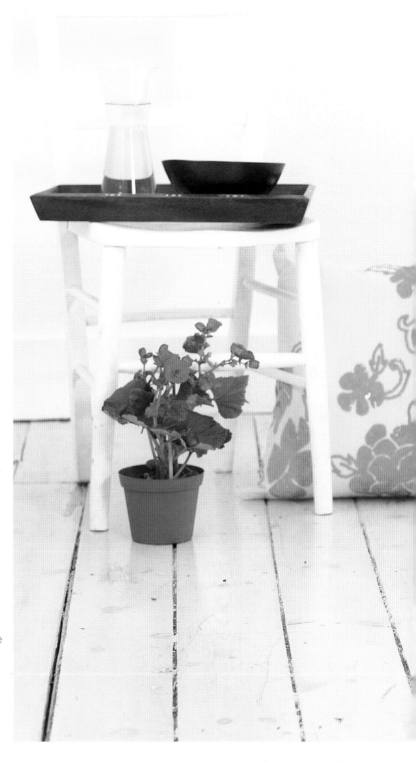

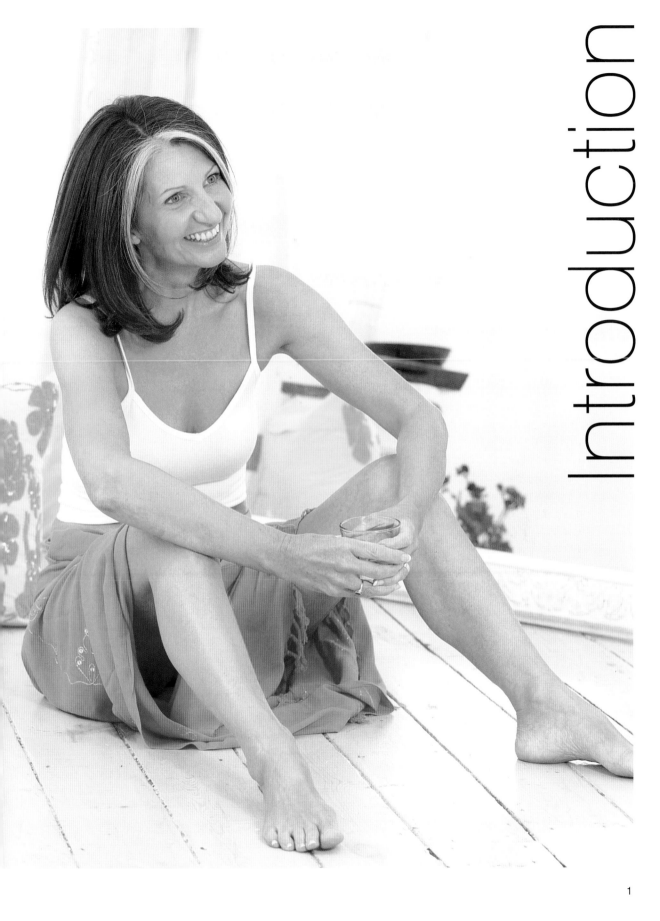

The Body Control Pilates® Way

I F YOU are looking for exercises for a perfect body, you need look no further than Body Control Pilates. Here is a proven method of body conditioning that is revolutionary in the way it can change you, inside and out. In essence it teaches you how to move well and exercise with thought and precision which, after all, is simply good common sense.

How long will it take you to feel the benefits? Joseph Pilates said, 'In ten sessions you will feel a difference, in twenty you will see a difference and in thirty you will have a new body.' And what a body! Not only will it be leaner and longer, it will also be more supple and stronger. *The Perfect Body the Pilates Way* is toned but not bulky, with strength coming from within. The benefits are almost endless:

- a firmer, flatter stomach
- improved posture
- greater flexibility
- toned arms and shoulders
- a defined waist
- firmer buttocks and thighs
- less cellulite
- more efficient breathing
- stronger back muscles
- better alignment
- better core strength
- improved balance
- better co-ordination
- greater bone density
- mobile joints
- improved circulation
- more energy
- stress relief
- an enhanced sex life
- a sense of wellbeing
- boosted immunity

Celebrities, dancers, and the rich and famous have known and enjoyed the benefits of Pilates for over eighty years. Joseph Pilates' original studio, which opened in the 1920s, was based in New York.
His clientele was drawn mainly from practitioners of the performing arts – dancers who used his exercises to supplement their traditional classical training or actors who wanted superb bodies that moved on the stage or movie set with ease and grace, for example. Among his regulars were Katherine Hepburn and Lauren Bacall. Following in their footsteps many illustrious stars have tried this unique form of exercise. To name a few:

- Uma Thurman
- Liz Hurley
- Sigourney Weaver
- Courteney Cox Arquette
- Jennifer Aniston
- Portia de Rossi
- Sarah Jessica Parker
- Stefanie Powers
- Tracy Ullman
- Jodie Foster
- Madonna
- Annie Lennox
- Sharon Stone

All these are beautiful, sexy women. But have you ever stopped to think what makes a woman possess sex appeal? It is not always perfect features or a perfect shape. The perfect body has more to do with a sense of confidence in yourself and making the most of what you've got. If you are comfortable with your body, have good body awareness and are relaxed, then you give out the right signals. How you dress, wear make-up, or what job you do, can add to or subtract from your sex appeal but, at the end of the day, you must be happy in your body. Pilates can help you know and enjoy your own body. As you learn the exercises you will learn about yourself.

Why Is Pilates So Effective?

PILATES WORKS on many levels and in a way that is totally unlike any other form of exercise. Fundamentally, the method aims to change the way you move, to re-educate your body's movement patterns, and to teach you how to move correctly. Joseph Pilates had no formal medical training but he recognized and understood good movement and good alignment. His sickly childhood had left him frail and weak, and in his search to improve his body he tried yoga, gymnastics, skiing, self-defence, dance, circus training and weight training. These different methods led him to devise his own programme of exercises; the hours he had dedicated to exploring other disciplines meant that he instinctively knew which exercises worked and which didn't.

How many of you have wondered why the sit-ups you are doing are not working? Why you still have not achieved the flat stomach you seek? Why your arms and thighs are still flabby despite frequent visits to the gym? The answer is that you are not working efficiently. Pilates gives you body awareness to understand how to make the most of your workout. It re-trains your body so that your movement patterns are sound and your posture is improved, which means that when you exercise you can target the right muscles. As long as you have bad movement patterns your workouts will only reinforce them: over-dominant muscles will carry on being over-active and become stronger, while weak muscles will remain weak. Furthermore, other fitness methods focus on the superficial muscles of the body while ignoring the all-important deeper postural muscles. Pilates works the other way round. First we teach you how to find and strengthen the deep core muscles, then we move on to build on that strength. This means that any changes which are made are based on strong foundations – giving you results that last.

We have included in this Pilates programme exercises for strength training using free weights and gravity resistance to build muscle into the body. If you then add three 20–30 minute sessions of aerobic activity a week, you have the perfect fitness plan.

Where Do You Start?

There are Eight Principles behind the Body Control Pilates Method:

- relaxation
- concentration
- alignment
- breathing
- centring
- co-ordination
- flowing movements
- stamina

Relaxation

This is the starting point for everyone learning Pilates. It may seem a strange way to begin an exercise routine, but our first priority is to make sure that everyday stress isn't brought into a session. By relaxed we do not mean collapsed but, rather, without unwanted tension, ready to move easily and freely. Learning how to recognize and release areas of tension is essential before you work out, because it helps prevent the use of the wrong muscles. We need to learn how to switch off over-active muscles otherwise they will continue to overwork, perpetuating unsound movement patterns. Most people hold tension around the back of the neck and the upper shoulders, but if a lot of time is spent sitting, the muscles at the front of the hips and the hamstrings also become very tight. We will be giving you gentle stretches to help ease out this tension.

The Relaxation Position on page 14 is a good way to start a session – you will notice that we also use it as the starting and finishing position for many of the exercises. As you advance in Pilates, however, you should be able to use any simple exercise to the same effect.

Concentration

Relaxation requires inner focus. Pilates is a mental and physical conditioning programme that should train both mind and body. It requires you to focus on each movement and develops your body's sensory feedback or kinaesthetic sense so that you know where you are in space and what you are doing with every part of your body for every second you are moving. Although the movements themselves may become automatic with time, you still have to concentrate because there is always a further level of awareness to reach. Use the exercises in this book to train your mind–body connection and you will find that you are far more body aware not just when you exercise but also in your daily activities. You will be able to concentrate better and be far more co-ordinated in your movements. Learn to listen to the natural intelligence of your body – it really does talk to you!

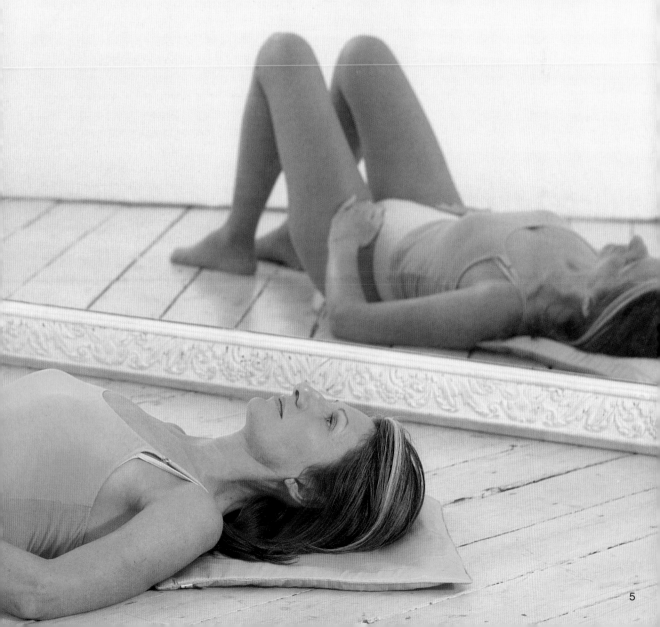

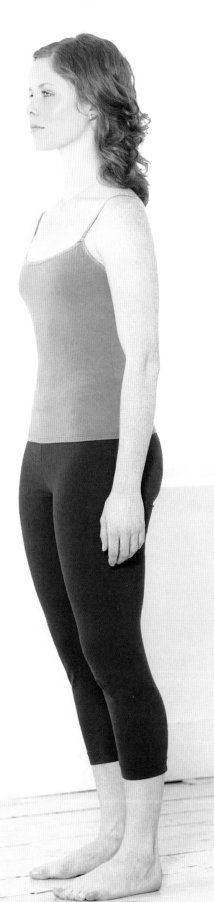

Alignment

By constantly reminding the body of how it should be standing, sitting or lying and by moving correctly, you can bring the body into better alignment – essential not only to restore muscle balance but also to looking good. Slouching is extremely unattractive – it makes you look shorter, fatter, round shouldered and even makes your breasts look droopy. Furthermore, if you exercise without concern for the correct position of the joints, you risk putting them under stress, which can lead to extra wear and tear and perhaps contribute to osteoarthritis. By placing your bones in the right place you get the right muscles working. In that way, you build the muscles so they will support the joint, not put it under stress. Most people do not realize that simply standing correctly works all the deep postural muscles.

Standing Correctly

This checklist should help you align your body correctly:

- Allow your head to go forward and up.
- Allow your neck to release.
- Relax your shoulder blades down into your back.
- Keep your breastbone soft.
- Keep your elbows open.
- Lengthen up through the spine.
- Check that the pelvis is in neutral (see page 15).
- Stand with the feet hip-distance apart and with the legs parallel.
- Release your knees.
- Keep the weight even on both feet – do not allow them to roll in or out.

Breathing

The Compass on page 15 is designed to help you find the correct neutral position of the pelvis and the spine. Once this is familiar in the Relaxation Position (see page 14), you should practise finding neutral while standing, sitting and lying on your side so that it becomes normal. All the exercises should be performed in this neutral position unless otherwise specified. Occasionally, if the muscles around the pelvis are very out of balance, you may find neutral difficult to maintain. If this is the case, consult a fully qualified Pilates practitioner, physiotherapist, chiropractic or osteopath. It is often necessary to work in what is the best neutral you can achieve, or use some support such as towels or flat pillows. Usually, after a few months, as the muscles begin to rebalance, neutral becomes more comfortable.

Improving your breathing is probably the single most dramatic difference you can make to your overall health – but it is the one thing we all take for granted. Few of us breathe efficiently, so we miss out on all that wonderful oxygen that can nourish and replenish every cell in the body. We may go to great expense to buy the latest oxygen-rich skin creams or, taking things to an extreme, may even spend time in oxygen tents – but the best results are to be had by simply learning to breathe more effectively, increasing the lung capacity, and using the lower as well as the upper lobes of the lungs. By taking the time to master lateral or thoracic breathing (see page 13), you can ultimately improve your hair, skin, nails, bones and your overall wellbeing. What's more, once this breathing becomes automatic you will reap the benefits every second of the day and night.

Centring: Creating a Girdle of Strength

Joseph Pilates had no formal medical training but he discovered that if he hollowed his navel back towards his spine, the lower back felt protected and he thus introduced the direction 'navel to spine' for all his exercises. He called the area between the hips and the ribcage the powerhouse and taught that all movement should originate from this strong centre. In so doing he was using the deep postural muscles to stabilize the spine – which modern physiotherapists now call core stability.

The key muscles are transversus abdominis, the deepest of your abdominal muscles, and multifidus a deep spinal muscle. The latest medical research indicates that the best stability comes when movement begins with the pelvic floor muscles and then engages the lower abdominals. This is why the direction 'zip up and hollow' is used in Body Control Pilates. As you breathe out you draw up the muscles of the pelvic floor and hollow the lower abdominal muscles back to the spine as if you are doing up an internal zip!

You will notice that the word 'hollow' is used to describe this movement. It is very important that you do not grip your abdominals tightly as this creates unnecessary tension and usually engages the wrong muscles. Stabilizing muscles should ideally be worked at less than 25 per cent of their full effort because they are postural muscles which need endurance. They work for you all day, every day! Once you have learned to create a strong centre, add movements such as rotation, flexion and extension. The exercises starting on page 21 will take you through this step by step.

Co-ordination

So, now you are relaxed, focused, aware, aligned, breathing efficiently (or learning to) and you have located and strengthened your deep core muscles, you are ready to add movement. Initially moving well isn't easy, but it soon becomes an automatic (grooved) movement – a muscle memory. Meanwhile, the actual process of learning this co-ordination is excellent mental and physical training, stimulating the two-way communication channel which feeds the brain good movement and sound recruitment patterns. Start with small motions and build up to more complicated combinations – the idea is to be constantly challenged. As beginners you need to keep your limbs close to you rather than risk losing your alignment and stability. Whatever exercise you are performing, the movements must be precisely executed with control. Frequent repetition of these sound movement patterns, making the right muscles work at the right length, at the right time in the right job, will start to change the way you move.

Flowing Movements

Pilates is all about natural movements performed smoothly, gracefully and with attention to detail. You will not be required to twist into awkward positions or to strain. The movements are generally slow, lengthening away from a strong centre, which gives you the opportunity to check alignment and focus on using the right muscles. Slow doesn't mean easy though – in fact it is harder to do an exercise slowly than quickly and it is also less easy to cheat!

Stamina

Finally, we wish to build endurance and stamina into the body. We can do this by challenging stability, working with longer levers (for example, an extended leg rather than a bent one), adding load with weights, using resistance or unstable surfaces. Many people complain of tiredness after a day on their feet, simply because standing badly is tiring: the ribcage is compressed and, as a consequence, the lungs are constricted. As you learn to open and lengthen the body, breathing becomes more efficient. All Pilates exercises are designed to encourage the respiratory, lymphatic and circulatory systems to function more effectively. As you become more proficient at the exercises and your muscles begin to work correctly, you will discover that your overall stamina improves dramatically. You will no longer be wasting energy by holding on to unnecessary tension or moving inefficiently. Think of a well-serviced car where the engine is tuned and the wheels aligned – it runs more efficiently, as will your body.

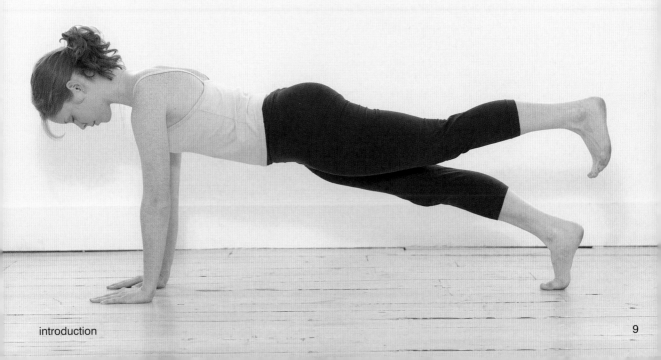

How to Prepare for Pilates

What You Need

- A straight-backed chair.
- A padded, non-slip mat or a yoga mat folded in half.
- A folded towel or a small, flat pillow.
- A plump pillow.
- A flatter, bedroom pillow.
- A tennis ball.
- A scarf, a long towel or a stretchband.
- Loose, comfortable clothing and bare feet.
- Hand-held weights of up to about 2.5 kg each weight (or easily held household items of the same weight).
- Ankle weights of up to about 1 kg each weight. Alternatively, use a pair of old tights (no holes!). Cut off the legs, tie a knot about 15 centimetres from the end, pour in uncooked rice or a similar dry substance of the correct weight and tie a knot about 15 centimetres from the other end. Repeat with the other leg of the tights and wrap around your ankles as needed.

Before You Begin

Prepare the space you are going to exercise in by making it warm, comfortable and free from distractions. Please do not exercise if:

- You are feeling unwell.
- You have just eaten a heavy meal.
- You have been drinking alcohol.
- You are in pain from an injury. Always consult your practitioner first, as rest may be needed before exercise.
- You have been taking painkillers, as they will mask any warning signs.
- You are undergoing medical treatment or are taking drugs. Again, you will need to consult your practitioner first.

> **Warning:** not all the exercises in this programme are suitable during pregnancy.

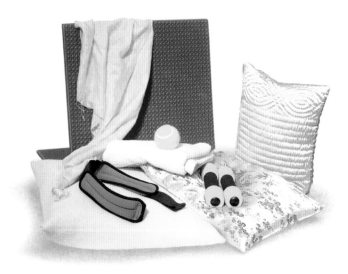

The Basics of Body Control Pilates®

Step by step we are now going to teach you the skills you will need to perform the exercises well. Once you have mastered one skill you can move on to the next, layering one on another. All our exercises are graded to help you to achieve this. You will find that learning one skill helps you learn the others. Remember how you felt on your first driving lesson? There was so much to remember: steering, clutch, gears, brake, mirrors, signals and so on. Then, all of a sudden, everything fell into place and you drove easily without having to think about each separate element. It's exactly the same with Pilates. At first you may despair of remembering to keep neutral, breathe wide and centre, but eventually it really does all come together and you will be ready to move on.

The basic skills you need to begin are breathing, good alignment and centring.

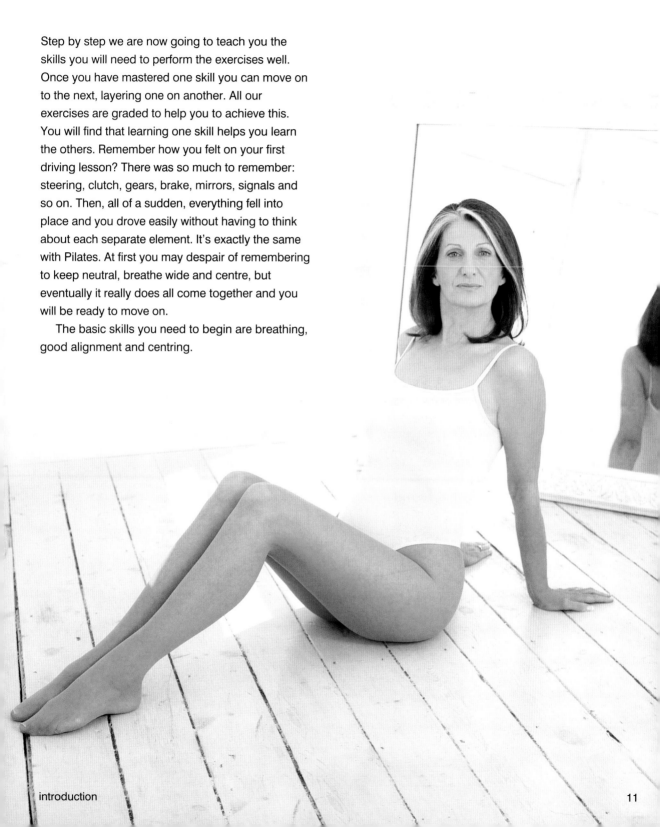

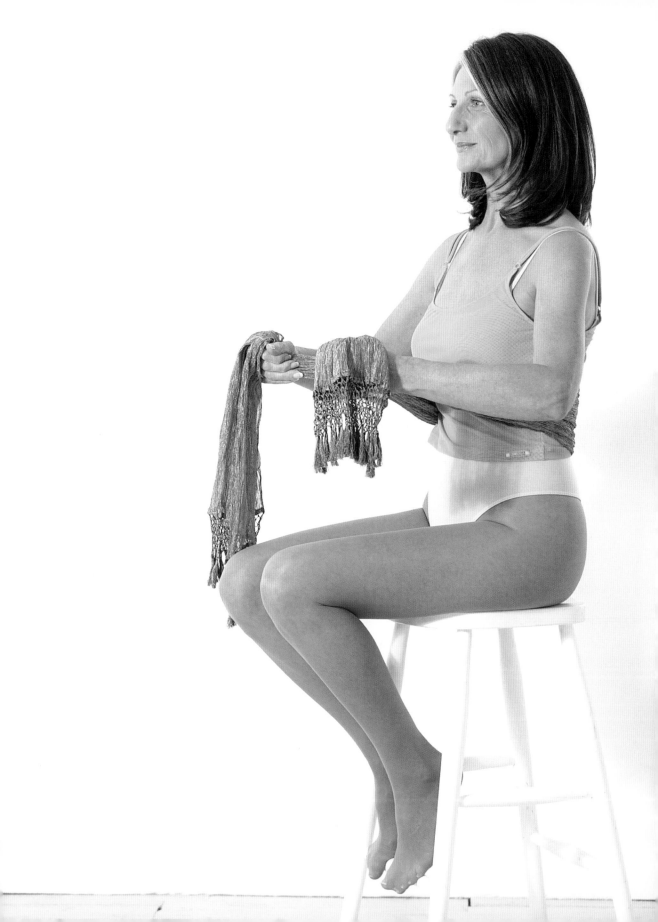

Breathing

Stand in front of a mirror and watch as you take a deep breath. Do your shoulders rise up around the ears? Perhaps your lower stomach expands when you breathe in? Most of us breathe inefficiently. Ideally, you should breathe wide and full expanding the ribcage by several centimetres. Think of a balloon expanding in all directions. By breathing this way, the volume of the chest cavity is increased and the capacity for oxygen intake is therefore also increased. It encourages maximum use of the lower part of the lungs as well.

This type of breathing – called thoracic or lateral breathing – makes the upper body more fluid and mobile. The lungs become like bellows, with the lower ribcage expanding wide as you breathe in and closing down as you breathe out. As you breathe in, your diaphragm automatically descends; you shouldn't block the descent of the diaphragm but encourage the movement to be widthways and into the back. The exercise below will help you learn thoracic breathing.

1   Sit or stand tall. Wrap a scarf or towel around your ribs, crossing it over at the front.
2   Holding the ends of the scarf and gently pulling it tight, breathe in and allow your ribs to expand the towel (watch that you do not lift the breastbone too high).
3   As you breathe out, you may gently squeeze the towel to help fully empty your lungs and relax the ribcage, allowing the breastbone to soften.

Breathing out, you will engage the pelvic floor muscles and hollow the abdomen (explained in Creating a Girdle of Strength on page 8) to give both lumbar and pelvic stability as you move. Ultimately you will need to keep these muscles engaged as you breathe in and out.

Never force the breath, it should flow naturally with the movement. Some people find this timing difficult at first, especially if you are used to other fitness regimes, but once you have mastered it, it makes sense.

As a general rule:

- Breathe in to prepare for a movement.
- Breathe out, zip up and hollow (see page 16) and move.
- Breathe in, still zipped, to recover.

Moving on the exhalation will enable you to relax into the stretch and prevent you from tensing. It also offers greater core stability at the hardest part of the exercise and safeguards against holding the breath, which can unduly stress the heart and lead to serious complications.

The Relaxation Position

We will be referring to this position throughout the book.

Equipment

A flat pillow or a folded towel (optional).

1 Lie on your back with a small towel or firm, flat pillow underneath your head, if necessary, to allow the back of the neck to lengthen.

2 Keep your feet parallel and hip-distance apart and your knees bent.

3 Rest your hands on the pelvis. Think of your elbows and shoulder blades opening out.

4 Release the neck, soften the breastbone and lengthen up through the spine.

5 The pelvis and spine should be in neutral (explained in Finding Neutral, see page 15), following their natural tilt and curve respectively.

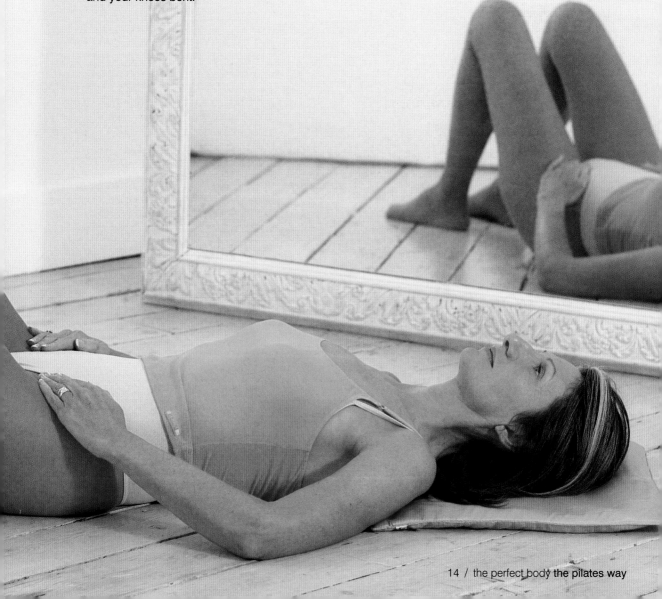

Alignment: Finding Neutral: The Compass

If you exercise with the pelvis and spine misplaced, you run the risk of creating muscle imbalances and putting stress on the spine itself. In Pilates, the aim is to have the pelvis and spine in their natural, neutral positions. To find neutral for these exercises, follow this sequence:

1 Lie in the Relaxation Position (see page 14).
2 Imagine you have a compass on your lower abdomen. The navel is north and the pubic bone south, with west and east on either side. Now try two incorrect positions in order to find the correct one.
3 Tilt your pelvis north. The pelvis will tuck under, the waist will flatten and the curve of the lower back is lost as your tailbone (coccyx) lifts off the floor. You will also grip the muscles around your hips and abdominals.
4 Next, carefully and gently move the pelvis in the other direction so that it tilts south (avoid this if you have a back injury). The low back will arch, the ribs will flare and the stomach will stick out. Come back to the starting position.
5 Aim for a neutral position between these two extremes. Go back to the image of the compass and think of the pointer as a spirit level. When you are in neutral, the pubic bone and the pelvic bones will be level. Your sacrum will rest squarely on the floor.

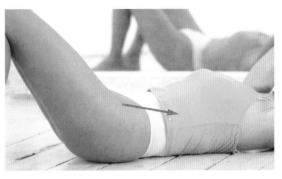

North

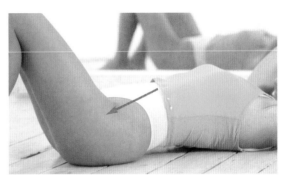

South

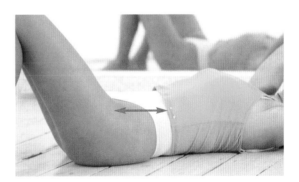

Neutral

Pilates Core Strength

Using your girdle of strength or powerhouse is at the centre of Pilates. You need to learn how to stabilize your lumbar spine, your pelvis and finally your shoulder blades and neck.

Centring: The Pelvic Elevator (*sitting*)

Aim

This exercise was created to isolate and engage the deep stabilizing muscles of the pelvis, pelvic floor and spine – transversus abdominis and multifidus. In order to achieve the best possible stability, you need to be able to contract the pelvic floor at the same time as hollowing the lower abdominals to engage tranversus abdominis. We call this zip up and hollow – it's as if you are doing up an internal zip.

It is not easy to isolate and engage the pelvic floor muscles and takes considerable concentration. They are the muscles of the vagina for women and of the urethra for both sexes (men should think about lifting their 'crown jewels'!). One way to help locate these muscles is to suck your thumb as you draw them up inside. It sounds crazy, but it works! You want to think about these muscles drawing together from side to side rather than from front to back, and then up a little (see below). Think of a camera shutter closing! At this stage we do not want you to engage the muscles around the anus, as it is too easy for the buttock muscles to kick in and substitute.

Once you have found the pelvic floor muscles, it should be easier to isolate tranversus abdominis. To engage these muscles correctly (at no more than 25 per cent) think of:

* hollowing
* scooping
* drawing back the abdominals towards the spine
* sucking in

Starting Position

Sit on an upright chair making sure that you are sitting square, with the weight even on both buttocks. Imagine that your pelvic floor is like the lift in a building and this exercise requires you to take the lift up to different floors.

Action

1 Breathe in wide and full into your back and sides, then lengthen up through the spine.
2 As you breathe out, draw up the muscles of your pelvic floor as if you are trying to prevent the flow of urine. Remember to draw them together from side to side rather than from front to back. Take the pelvic lift up to the first floor of the building. This is as far as you need to go to engage the muscles to zip up and hollow.
3 Breathe in and release the lift back to the ground floor.

It is useful though to feel what it is like to pull up the pelvic floor further so . . .

4 Breathe out and take the lift up to the second floor of the building.
5 Breathe in and release.
6 Breathe out and take the lift up to the third floor. Notice how when you do this, the six-pack muscles (rectus abdominis) of your abdomen automatically engage.
7 Breathe in and relax.

Watchpoints

* When you reached the first floor, you should have felt the deep lower abdominals engage. This is transversus coming into play. By starting the action from underneath, you encourage the six-pack muscle to stay quiet. If you were to take the lift all the way to the top floor, you would probably be engaging the muscles at over 30 per cent, causing the six-pack muscle to take over – so keep the action low and gentle.
* Do not allow the buttock muscles to join in.
* Keep your jaw relaxed.
* Don't take your shoulders up to the top floor too – keep them down and relaxed.
* Try not to grip around your hips.
* Keep the pelvis and spine quite still.

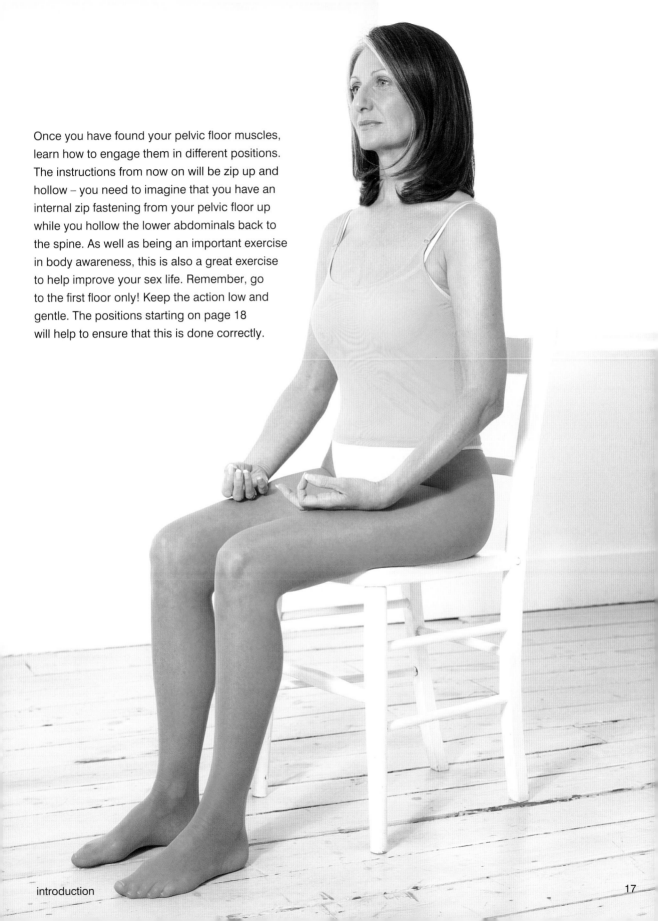

Once you have found your pelvic floor muscles, learn how to engage them in different positions. The instructions from now on will be zip up and hollow – you need to imagine that you have an internal zip fastening from your pelvic floor up while you hollow the lower abdominals back to the spine. As well as being an important exercise in body awareness, this is also a great exercise to help improve your sex life. Remember, go to the first floor only! Keep the action low and gentle. The positions starting on page 18 will help to ensure that this is done correctly.

introduction

Stabilizing on All Fours

Try this wearing just your underwear, with a mirror underneath you. You can check to see if your six-pack remains quiet.

Starting Position

Kneel on all fours with your hands beneath your shoulders and your knees beneath your hips. Have the top of your head lengthening away from your tailbone and your pelvis in neutral. It's useful to imagine a small puddle of water resting in the small of your back. This helps you to stay neutral.

Action

1 Breathe in to prepare.
2 Breathe out and zip up and hollow. Your back should not move.
3 Breathe in and release.
4 Now, try to keep zipped while breathing in and out.

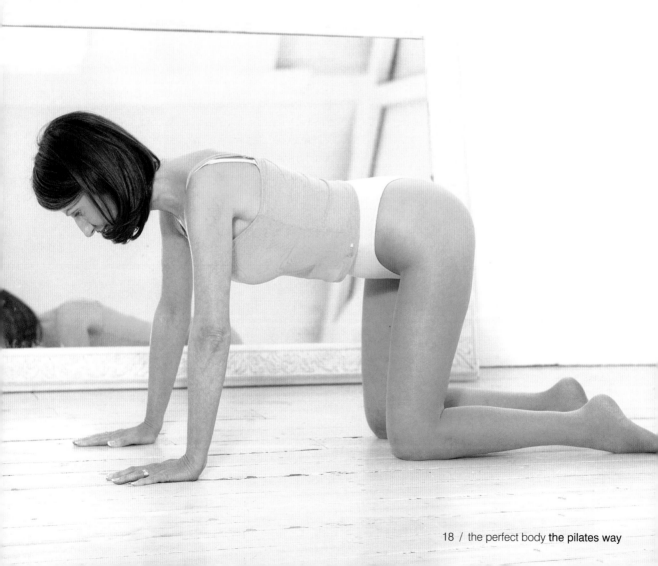

Stabilizing in Prone Lying

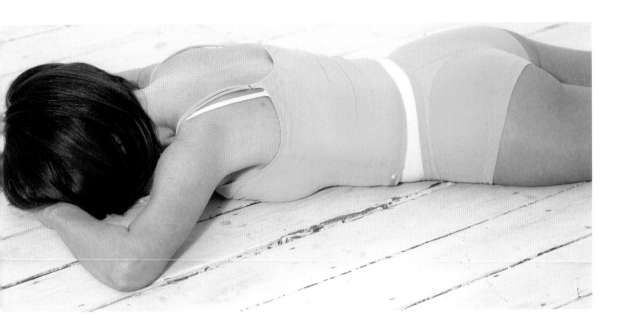

This, then, is your strong centre. For most of the exercises, you will be asked to zip up and hollow before and during your movements, lengthening away from a strong centre.

Equipment
A small, flat cushion (optional).

Starting Position
Lie face down, resting your forehead on your folded hands. Open the shoulders out and relax the upper back (use a small, flat cushion under your abdomen if your low back is uncomfortable). Your legs are shoulder-distance apart and relaxed.

Action
1 Breathe in to prepare.
2 Breathe out, zip up and hollow, drawing the lower abdominals away from the floor.
3 Imagine there is a precious egg just above the pubic bone that must not be crushed. Do not tighten the buttocks. There should be no movement in the pelvis or the spine.
4 Breathe in and release.
5 Once again, try to stay zipped as you breathe in and out.

Stabilizing in the Relaxation Position

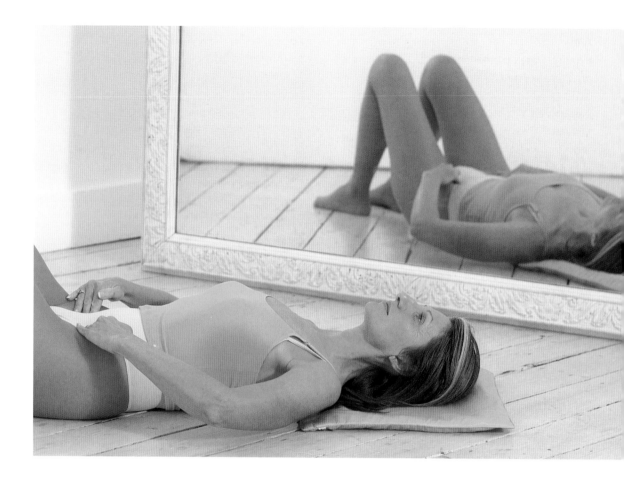

Starting Position

Lie in the Relaxation Position (see page 14). Check that your pelvis is in neutral. Now gently feel your lower abdominals, a few inches in and down from your pelvic bones.

Action

1 Breathe in to prepare and lengthen the spine.
2 Breathe out and zip up and hollow.
3 Do not allow the pelvis to tuck under. Do not push into the spine. Keep your tailbone on the floor and lengthening away.
4 Now breathe normally, staying zipped and hollowed. Take six breaths.

You must be careful not to tuck the pelvis under (tilting north). If you do, you will lose your neutral position. It also means that other muscles – the six-pack muscles and the hip flexors – are doing the work instead of the transversus muscle. If you are comfortable with your hand under your waist, check to see if you are pushing into the spine. Once you have learned to create a strong centre, you can add limb movements and then others such as rotation, flexion and extension.

Pelvic Stability – Leg Slides, Drops, Folds and Turnout

Aim

Having mastered breathing, correct alignment and the creation of a strong centre, learn how to add movement co-ordinating all this. It isn't easy to begin with, but it soon becomes automatic. Meanwhile, the process of learning this co-ordination is fabulous mental and physical training, stimulating that two-way communication between the brain and the muscles.

Start with small movements, then build up to more complicated combinations. Below are four movements to practise, all of them requiring you to keep the pelvis completely still. A useful image is to imagine that you have a set of car headlamps on your pelvis, shining at the ceiling. The beam should be fixed, rather than mimicking searchlights. You can vary which exercises you practise each session but the starting position is the same for all three.

Starting Position

Lie in the Relaxation Position (see page 14). Check that your pelvis is in neutral, your tailbone down and lengthening away, then place your hands on your pelvic bones to check for unwanted movement.

Action for Leg Slides

1 Breathe in wide and full to prepare.
2 Breathe out and zip up and hollow.
3 Sliding one leg away along the floor in line with your hips, keep the lower abdominals engaged and the pelvis still, stable and in neutral.
4 Breathe into your lower ribcage while you return the leg to the bent position, trying to keep the stomach hollow. If you cannot yet breathe in and maintain a strong centre, take an extra breath and return the leg on the out breath.
5 Repeat five times with each leg.

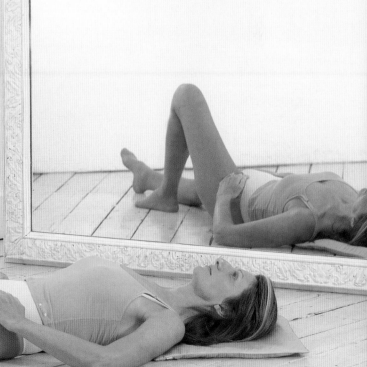

Action for Knee Drops

1 Breathe in wide and full to prepare.
2 Breathe out, zip up and hollow, and allow one knee to open slowly to the side. Go only as far as the pelvis can stay still.
3 Breathe in, still zipped and hollowed, and return the knee to centre.
4 Repeat five times with each leg.

Action for Knee Folds

With this movement it is particularly useful to feel that the muscles stay scooped and do not bulge while you fold the knee in. Very gently feel the muscles engage as you zip up and hollow.

1 Breathe in wide and full to prepare.
2 Breathe out, zip up and hollow, then fold the left knee up. Think of the thighbone dropping down into the hip and anchoring there.
3 Do not lose your neutral pelvis – the tailbone stays down – and do not rely on the other leg to stabilize you. Imagine your foot is on a cream cake and you don't want to press down on it.
4 Breathe in and hold.
5 Breathe out, still zipped and hollowed as you slowly return the foot to the floor.
6 Repeat five times with each leg.

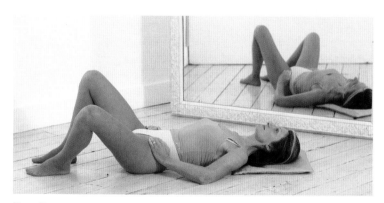

Knee Drops

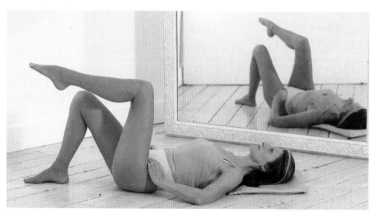

Knee Folds

Action for Turning out the Leg

This next action involves turning the leg out from the hip and is a preparation for exercises such as the Passé Développés on page 156 where the legs are held in a turned-out position. It works the deep gluteal muscles, especially gluteus medius which is one of the main stabilizing muscles of the pelvis.

1 Breathe in wide and full to prepare.
2 Breathe out, zip up and hollow then fold the left knee up. Think of the thighbone dropping down into the hip and anchoring there.
3 Breathe in and then out, zip up and hollow and turn the left leg out from the hip bringing the foot to touch the right knee if possible. Keep the knee above the hip.
4 Do not allow the pelvis to tilt or twist or turn, keep it central and stable (remember the headlamps should be glued to the ceiling).
5 Breathe in and then out, and zip up and hollow as you reverse the movement to return the foot to the floor.
6 Repeat five times to each side.

Watchpoints

- Remember that you are trying to avoid even the slightest movement of the pelvis. It helps to think of the waist being long and even on both sides as you make the movement.
- Try to keep your neck and jaw released throughout.

> **Warning:** please take advice if you suffer from sciatica.

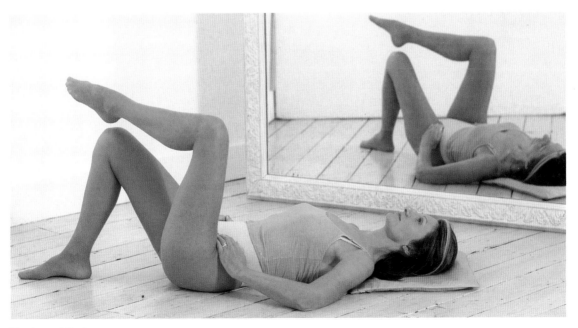

Turning out the Leg

Scapular Stability: The Dart *Stage One*

The final part of our girdle of strength lesson involves learning how to stabilize the shoulder blades and move the upper body correctly, with good mechanics. For this, you need to find the trapezius and serratus anterior muscles that set the shoulder blades down into the back, placing the shoulder joint itself in just the right position to allow the arm to move freely and easily. To find these muscles, try this exercise:

Equipment
A flat pillow or a folded towel (optional).

Starting Position
Lie face down (you can place a pillow or towel under your forehead to allow you to breathe), with your arms down by your sides and your palms facing your body. Your neck is long and your legs together, relaxed and parallel, toes softly pointed.

Action
1. Breathe in to prepare and lengthen through the spine, tucking in your chin gently as if you were holding a ripe peach beneath it.
2. Breathe out, zip up and hollow, and slide your shoulder blades down into your back, lengthening your fingers down towards your feet.
3. The top of your head stays lengthening away from you too.
4. Keep looking straight down at the floor. Do not tip your head back.
5. Breathe in and feel the length of the body from the tips of your toes to the top of your head.
6. Breathe out, still zipping, and release.

Watchpoints
- Keep hollowing the lower abdominals.
- Do not strain the neck – it should feel released as your shoulders engage down into your back. Think of a swan's neck growing out from between its wings.
- Keep your feet on the floor.
- Stop if you feel at all uncomfortable in the low back (you may find placing a flat pillow under your stomach helps). This exercise can also be done with the feet hip-width apart and the thigh and buttock muscles relaxed.

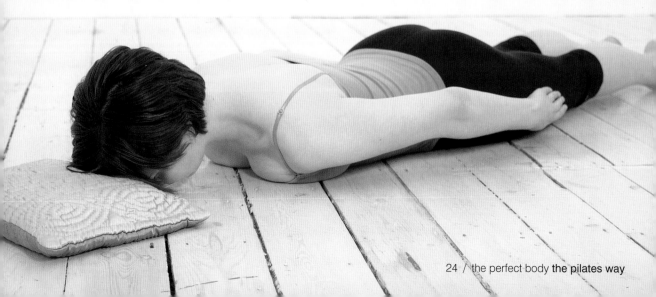

Floating Arms

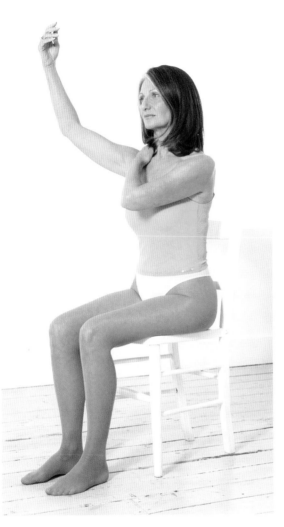

The muscles that you felt pulling your shoulder blades down into your back in the previous exercise are the stabilizing muscles. Now that you have located them, try to feel them working in this exercise.

Aim
To learn correct upper-body mechanics.

Starting Position
Sit on a chair or adopt the standing position described on page 6. Place your right hand on your left shoulder. Your hand checks that the upper part of your trapezius muscle remains quiet. Very often this part will overwork, so think of it staying soft and released, while the lower trapezius below your shoulder blades works to set the shoulder blades down into your back. As your arm rises above shoulder height, your shoulder blades will glide and coil outwards around the ribcage.

Action
1 Breathe in to prepare and lengthen up through the spine, letting the neck relax.
2 Breathe out and zip up and hollow. Slowly begin to raise the arm, reaching wide out of the shoulder blade like a bird's wing. Think of the hand as leading the arm – the arm follows the hand as it floats upwards.
3 Rotate the arm so that the palm opens to the ceiling as the arm reaches shoulder level. Try to keep the shoulder under your hand as still as possible and the shoulder blades dropping down into your back for as long as possible.
4 Breathe in as you lower the arm to your side.
5 Repeat three times with each arm.

Watchpoints
- Keep a sense of openness in the upper body.
- Do not allow your upper body to shift to the side, keep centred.

The Starfish *The Upper Body – Stage One*

Aim

To combine everything you have learnt so far.

Starting Position

Lie in the Relaxation Position (see page 14), but with your arms down by your sides.

Action

1 Breathe wide into your lower ribcage to prepare.
2 Breathe out, zip up and hollow, and start to take one arm back in a backstroke movement as if to touch the floor behind your head. You may not be able to touch the floor comfortably so only move the arm as far as you are happy to do so.
3 Do not force the arm – keep it soft and open with the elbow bent. Think of the shoulder blade drawing down into your back. The ribs stay down and calm. Do not allow the back to arch at all.
4 Breathe in as you return the arm to your side.
5 Repeat five times with each arm.

Note: not everyone can touch the floor behind them without arching the upper back, so do not strain. It is better to keep the back down than force the arm to the floor.

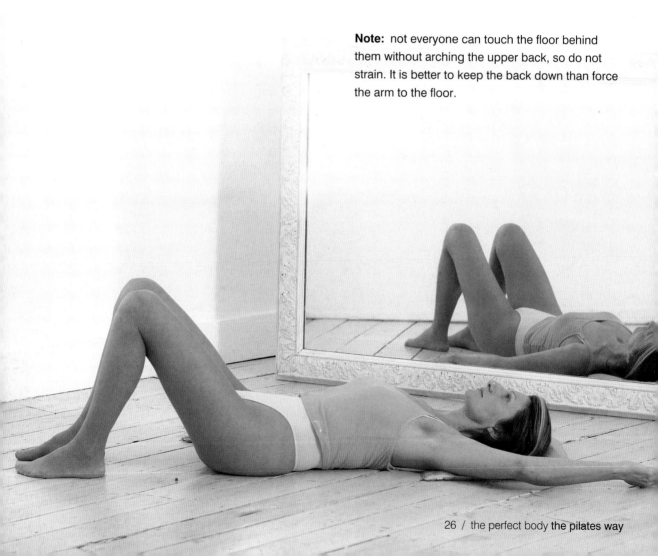

The Full Starfish *Stage Two*

Now we are going to co-ordinate the opposite arm and leg movement, away from our strong centre. Although this looks simple, it is a sophisticated movement pattern, using all the skills of good movement learnt so far.

Starting Position
Lie in the Relaxation Position (see page 14), with your arms down by your sides.

Action
1 Breathe in wide and full to prepare.
2 Breathe out and zip up and hollow.
  Slide the left leg away along the floor
  in a line with your hips and take the right
  arm above you in a backstroke movement.
3 Keep the pelvis completely neutral, stable
  and still and the stomach muscles engaged.
4 Keep a sense of width and openness in the
  upper body and shoulders, and think of the
  shoulder blades setting down into your back.
5 Breathe in, still zipped and hollowed, and return
  the limbs to the preparation position.
6 Repeat five times alternating arms and legs.

Watchpoints
• Do not be tempted to overreach –
  the girdle of strength must stay in place.
• Slide the leg in a line with the hip.
• Keep your actions natural and flowing.
• Keep your ribcage down.

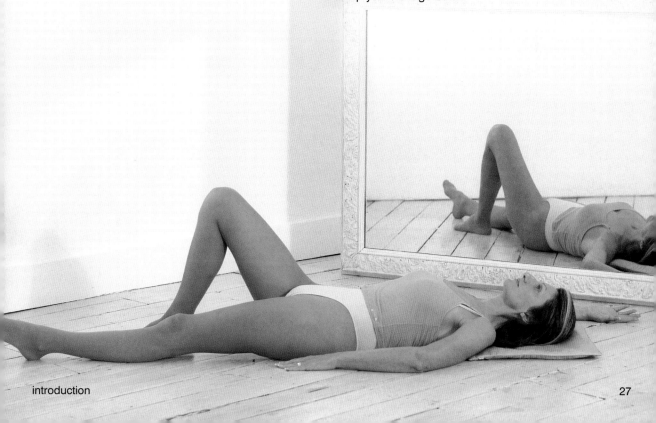

Neck Rolls and Chin Tucks

Aim

This exercise will release tension from the neck, freeing the cervical spine. It also uses the deep stabilizers of the neck, the deep neck flexors, and lengthens the neck extensors at the back of the neck. Please take note that this is a subtle movement – you should tuck your chin in gently.

Equipment

A flat pillow (optional).

Starting Position

Lie in the Relaxation Position (see page 14) with your hands resting on your lower abdomen. Only use a flat pillow if you are uncomfortable without one (your head will roll better if you do not have one).

Action

1 Release your neck and jaw, allowing your tongue to widen at its base. Keep the neck nicely lengthened, and soften your breastbone. Allow the shoulder blades to widen and melt into the floor.
2 Now, allow your head to roll slowly to one side.
3 Bring it back to the centre and over to the other side, taking your time.
4 When the neck feels free, bring the head to the centre and gently tuck your chin in, as if holding a ripe peach under it (you do not want to crush the delicate skin). Keep your head on the floor, lengthening out of the back of the neck.
5 Return the head to the centre.
6 Repeat the rolling to the side and chin tuck eight times.

Watchpoints

- Do not force the head or neck – just let it roll naturally.
- Do not lift the head off the floor when you tuck the chin in.

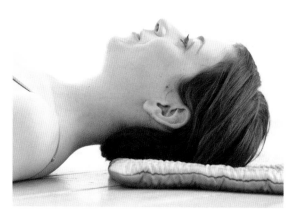

Starting position

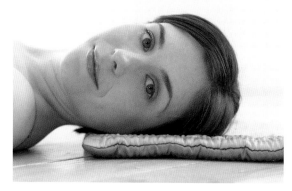

Neck Rolls

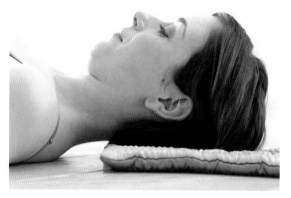

Chin Tucks

Pointing

Aim

To learn how to point and flex the feet,
while still maintaining good alignment
in the rest of the legs.

By pointing the foot or toes, we intend that you
softly point them. A very common mistake is that
you over-point and the foot then becomes sickled
(like a sickle). Instead, we want you to keep the
front of the foot long and make sure that the toes
do not curl under.

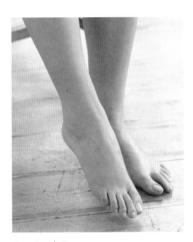

Good point

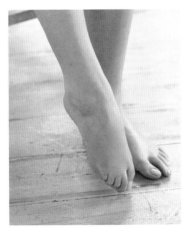

Bad point

Flexing

By flexing the foot, we intend that you push your
heel away from your face. The toes will come up
towards your face but, again, they do not curl over.
Keep them long, the heel lengthening away

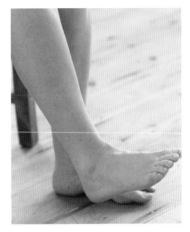

Good flex

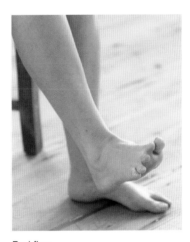

Bad flex

introduction

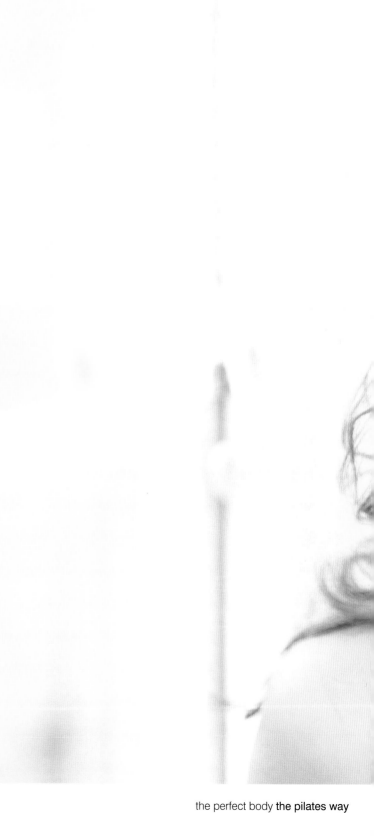

IN TODAY'S self-conscious and appearance-obsessed society, it seems that beautiful skin is no longer a luxury but something every woman is expected to achieve. Good skin is the most visible indicator of beauty and health. Few are born with it, most of us have to work for it; but anyone who has stood face to face with a supermodel would be able to reassure you that even the most beautiful women in the world have flaws. Putting the perfection into your complexion should be simple. Nothing more is needed than a basic understanding of how and why your skin behaves as it does; a few changes to the way you eat, drink and live; and, maybe the most overlooked element, learning to enjoy your skincare routine. The pay-off will be not only looking younger and healthier, but also the sense of wellbeing brought on by making time for yourself.

Face and Neck

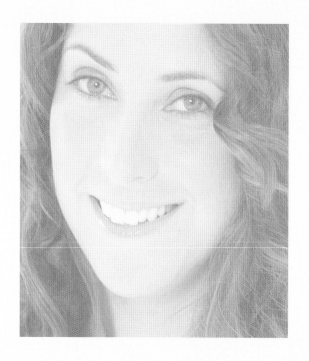

Smile Therapy

Did you know that when you meet someone, the first thing they will look at after your eyes is your teeth? The importance of an attractive smile and therefore good oral hygiene has grown massively in the public consciousness during the past few years. With the dazzling smiles of famous faces always in view in magazines and on television, the cult of celebrity has certainly played a large part in this. Bright, white teeth instantly make you look younger and healthier, giving you a confidence boost in the process. 'It's been called the dental facelift,' says Dr Malcom Torz of the London Day Surgery, who is a leading exponent of BriteSmile, the brilliant one-hour bleaching technique favoured by stars such as Catherine Zeta Jones and Heather Locklear. 'We live in a "now" society. We want what works quickest and best, so people have started to realize that sometimes cosmetic procedures can be a waste of time and money if you have terrible teeth.' Daily flossing and brushing for at least three minutes will establish good oral hygiene to combat cavities, gum disease and bad breath. If you like to eat fruit for breakfast you should know that brushing your teeth within an hour of eating acidic food can leave the protective enamel that coats them vulnerable to erosion. It is best to clean your teeth either before you eat fruit or to wait for an hour afterwards.

Exercises for the Face and Neck

How can Pilates exercises help improve the appearance of your face? In many ways. The Pilates Method does not have face exercises per se. However, anyone who takes up the method knows that one of the first things that happens soon after starting Pilates is that friends ask you, 'Have you had a holiday?' The time you spend on yourself in your Pilates session whether it be with a teacher or on your own at home is precious. As you focus on your breathing, as you calm your mind and concentrate on your flowing movements, your body responds accordingly. The worries of the outside world evaporate as you zip up and hollow, and try to maintain a neutral pelvis. In the meantime, the exercises stimulate your circulatory, respiratory and lymphatic systems. Blood flows freely, carrying oxygen to every cell, toxins are eliminated, your adrenal glands (situated above your kidneys and responsible for much of your wellbeing) thrive on the relaxation and gentle exercise. Endorphins are released – you feel good. No wonder you look as if you've had a two-week break. And, as you gradually tone your body, miraculously your cheekbones appear, your skin becomes clearer, the lines fainter. As you exercise, blood flows to your face, especially with the inverted exercises such as Roll Downs on page 82 or the Wall Exercises on pages 162–5. All this has the same effect as a good facial.

Evidence has shown that some forms of fitness regime can cause wrinkles because many of us screw up our faces as we perform the exercises and push ourselves to the limit. This is never the case in Pilates where the emphasis is on release of tension.

As you do these exercises (in fact as you do all the exercises in the book) concentrate on smoothing and softening the facial muscles. Allow your tongue to widen at its base and rest comfortably at the bottom of your mouth.

Think how elegant a ballet dancer is; this is in part due to good head, neck and shoulder alignment which is fundamental to Pilates training. Every time we ask you to lengthen up through the spine, release the neck and relax the shoulders we are taking you a step nearer to this natural grace.

Neck Turns, Crescents and Stretches (*beginners*)

These will gently ease out tension from the neck and shoulders.

It is good to take your neck through these movements to keep it supple and fully mobile.

Starting Position

Sit or stand tall. Your feet are on the floor hip-width apart and parallel. Have your hands resting softly on your knees, palms down.

Action

1 Breathe in wide and full and lengthen through the spine.

2 Breathe out and slowly turn your head to one side. Keep lengthening up through the top of your head; your shoulder blades stay down in your back.

3 Breathe in and return the head to the centre.

4 Breathe out and take your head the other way.

5 Repeat this three times to each side, then . . .

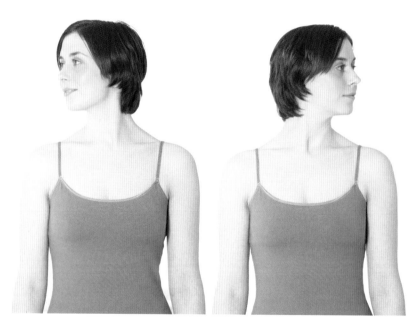

Neck Turns

6 Slowly drop your chin on to your chest, making sure that you do not round your upper back as you do so. Keep your shoulder blades down into your back.

7 Gently roll your chin in a quarter circle to the right, eventually bringing it up to look directly over your right shoulder.

8 Now, reverse the action tracing a semi-circle rolling down and up until you are looking over your left shoulder.

9 Repeat this gentle rolling action five times to each side, then . . .

10 Sit on your left hand with the palm upward.

11 Breathe in wide and full and lengthen through the spine.

12 Breathe out and slowly and gently tilt your right ear down towards your right shoulder. Feel the stretch on the left side of your neck – it should be comfortable.

13 Hold the stretch for a few moments until the tension releases, breathing normally.

14 Come out of the stretch very slowly.

15 Repeat on the other side.

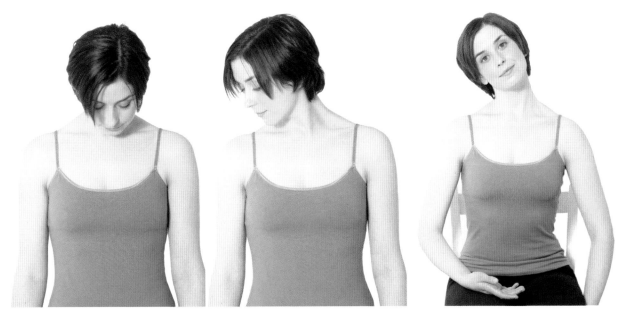

Crescents   Stretches

CAROLE MAGGIO'S FACERCISE®

Facercise® is the market leader in 'natural facelifts', and has helped thousand of men and women improve their looks without surgery. Using scientifically designed precision exercises that work directly on the facial muscles, dramatic results can be achieved in only six days.

Neck and Chin Toner

Great for firming the chin, neck and jawline, this exercise works and strengthens the platysma muscle. It can greatly reduce double chins and, in some cases, can almost make them invisible.

1 Sit tall and straight with your chin held high. Close your lips and smile strongly (without your teeth showing). Place one hand at the base of the throat over the collar bone and pull down slightly on the skin with a firm grip.
2 Tilt your head back and release to feel a strong pull on the chin and neck muscles. Tilt head backwards, count to three and then return to a normal head position. Repeat thirty-five times.

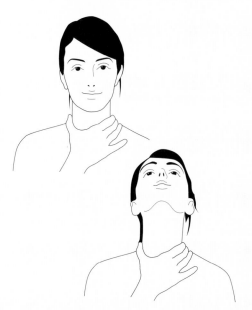

Lip Shaper

By working the obicularis oris muscle around the mouth, the Lip Shaper enlarges the lips and smooths out lines above the upper lip.

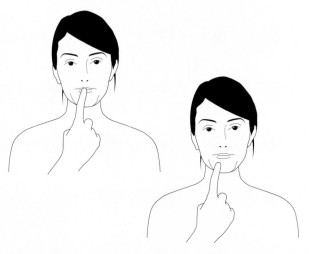

1 This can be done sitting up or lying down. Press your lips together. Do not purse your lips or clench your teeth. Tap the centre of your lips with your index finger. Visualize crushing a pencil between your lips.
2 Slowly pull your finger away from the centre of your lips. Visualize the pencil growing longer. Draw the energy point out and lengthen your imaginary pencil until you feel the burn. When you feel the burn pulse your finger up and down rapidly for a count of thirty. Release the lactic acid by blowing put through pressed lips.

Lip Shaper Tip Do the Lip Shaper twice a day to plump up thin lips. This is a fabulous exercise for people who hold stress and tension in their mouth area.

Eye Enhancer

The Eye Enhancer exercises the obicularis oculi muscle, which opens and closes the eye and surrounds it entirely. This exercise pumps blood into the eye area, strengthening the eyelids, reducing under-eye puffiness, lifting under-eye hollows and, in effect, enlarges the eye socket, giving you a more wide-awake, bright-eyed look.

1 You can perform this exercise lying down or in a sitting position. Place your middle fingers between your brows, above the bridge of your nose. Place your index fingers with light pressure at your outer eye corners (not allowing your eyebrows to furrow or wrinkle). Make a strong squint up with the lower eyelid. Feel the outer eye muscle pulse. Squint up and release ten times while focusing on the muscle pulsing each time.

2 Hold the squint and squeeze your eyes tightly shut, keeping your buttocks tight, and count to forty. It's very important to keep your eyes closed tightly and your buttocks clenched as you count.

Cheek Developer Tip
If you experience an ache in the jaw area, you are using your jaw to smile and release the cheeks, not your upper lip. Use only the upper lip, pressing down against the teeth. To alleviate an ache, blow between your lips.

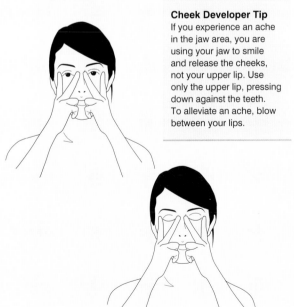

Cheek Developer

The Cheek Developer exercises the buccinator muscle. This is the rounded top part, or 'apple' of the cheek. The exercise also works the obicularis oris, which is the circular muscle surrounding the mouth. It lifts and enlarges the cheeks and removes hollows from under the eyes.

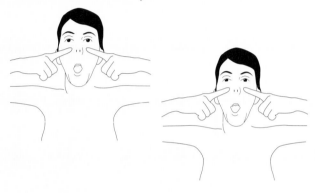

1 The exercise can be performed while sitting, moving or lying down. Imagine a dot in the centre of your upper lip. Imagine another dot in the centre of your lower lip. Open your mouth and pull the two dots apart. This should form a strong oval shape. Hold this shape firmly in place, keeping the upper lip pressing down against the teeth. Place your index fingers lightly on top of each cheek (the apple).

2 Smile with your mouth corners and then release the corners. Push the energy up under the cheek muscles and repeat this movement thirty-five times in quick succession. Use your mind–muscle connection to visualize pushing the muscle up under the cheek each time you smile. You should feel your cheeks moving as you do this exercise. To enhance the movement, you can tighten and release your buttocks each time you smile and release your mouth corners. This helps you to push the cheeks harder.

For more exercises and further information on the transforming effects of this comprehensive facial exercise programme, consult Carole Maggio's **The New Facercise**® *Give Yourself a Natural Facelift* www.facercise.com

Eating for Healthy Skin

The food we eat affects how good our skin looks. A radiant, blemish-free complexion relies on eating a wide variety of vitamins, minerals and other nutrients. Dermatologists and nutritionists agree that as often as possible, these should come from whole foods rather than from supplements so, to keep skin in optimum condition, regularly include these foods in your diet.

Five Foods for a Beautiful Complexion

Tomatoes

Packed with antioxidants including vitamins C and E and lycopene, tomatoes help protect the skin against damage by free radicals. Triggered by sun, smoking, stress and pollution, free radicals form inside us, breaking down the collagen and elastin fibres that keep skin plump and firm. By counteracting them, antioxidants help ensure skin doesn't age prematurely. Tomatoes also contain beta-carotene, which the body converts to vitamin A, essential for renewing the skin's cells.

Avocados

Avocados are high in monounsaturated fat, which is crucial for a soft, smooth complexion. They are also rich in vitamin E, a powerful antioxidant and wrinkle-fighter with the ability to help heal skin and minimize scarring. The vitamin B6 in avocados is a key ingredient in building the proteins used for the repair and renewal of body tissues including the skin.

Blackberries

Another excellent source of the vitamin C needed for healthy skin and to fight infections, blackberries also contain useful amounts of fibre for healthy digestion, as well as the flavonoid anthocyanidin, a phytochemical thought to have stronger anti-inflammatory and antioxidant properties than vitamin E.

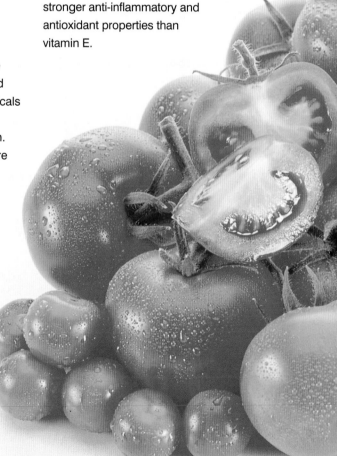

Feed Your Face

Packed with the antioxidants and nutrients that promote clear, glowing skin, try the vibrant recipes on pages 40 and 41.

Sesame Seeds

These tasty seeds are rich in the nutrients that maintain our tissue and muscle function. Sesame seeds contain B vitamins which help repair damaged cells and essential fatty acids which build strong skin and help keep it hydrated by balancing the body's fluid level. Sesame seeds are also full of zinc, which plays many important roles, particularly in healing. Zinc prompts the body to utilize vitamin C, it works as an anti-inflammatory and ensures smooth cell reproduction to help combat breakouts.

Kiwi Fruit

Weight for weight, kiwi fruit contain almost twice as much vitamin C as oranges – one large kiwi fruit will provide you with your complete recommended intake for the day. Vitamin C is essential if the skin is to produce the collagen that makes it strong and healthy. It is also an anti-inflammatory and fights infection, making kiwi fruit beneficial for anyone with an easily irritated or spot-prone complexion.

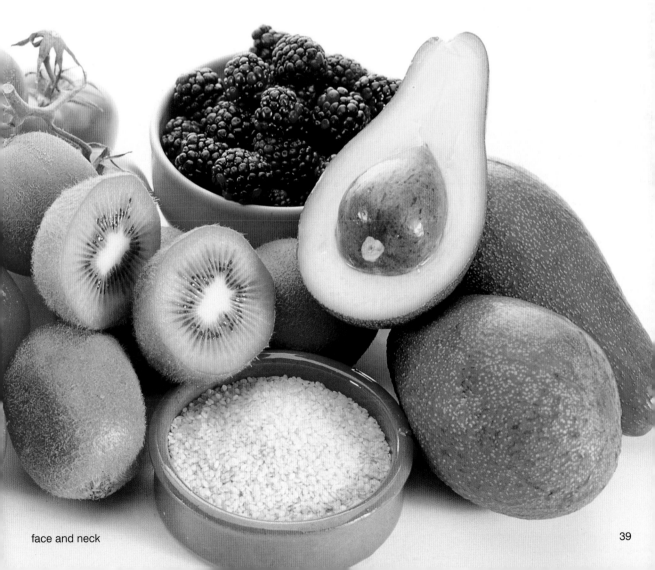

face and neck

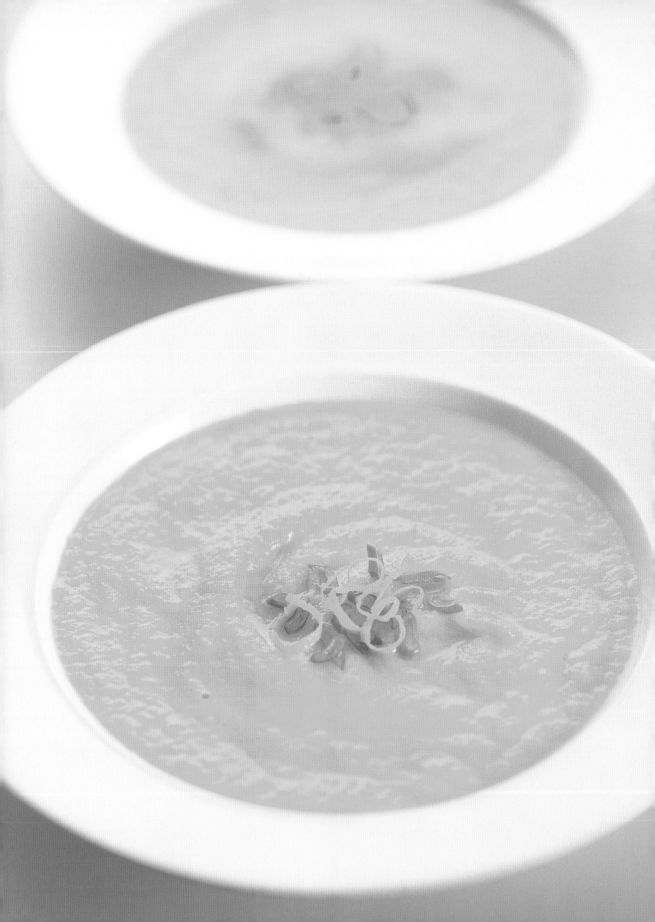

Carrot, Orange and Ginger Soup

Preparation time: **15 minutes**
Cooking time: **40 minutes**
Serves: **4–6**

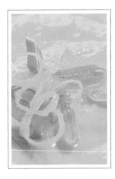

2 tbsp olive oil
1 medium onion, peeled and finely chopped
1 clove garlic, crushed or finely chopped
5cm piece fresh root ginger, finely chopped
600g carrots, peeled and roughly chopped
700ml vegetable stock
juice and zest of 2 large oranges
salt and freshly ground black pepper
spring onions, finely chopped

Heat the oil in a large pan, add the onion, garlic and ginger and cook over a medium heat for 3–4 minutes. Add the carrots and continue to cook for a further 5 minutes, stirring occasionally.

Add the stock, orange juice, zest and seasoning, then bring to the boil. Reduce the heat, cover and simmer for 30 minutes or until the carrots are soft.

Transfer the soup to a food processor or liquidizer and purée until smooth.

Return to the pan and reheat gently.

Ladle the soup into serving bowls and garnish with the spring onions.

Mixed Berry Brulée

Preparation time: **10 minutes, plus 2 hours chilling**
Cooking time: **Up to 3 minutes**
Serves: **4**

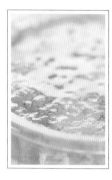

125g blueberries

125g raspberries

125g strawberries, hulled and roughly chopped

4 passion fruit, seeds removed

300ml Greek-style yoghurt

125g soft brown sugar

Mix the fruit in a large bowl and divide between 4 ovenproof ramekin dishes. Spoon the yoghurt over the fruit and chill for at least 2 hours.

Sprinkle the sugar over the yoghurt and place under a pre-heated, hot grill until the sugar caramelizes. Transfer to the fridge and chill until needed.

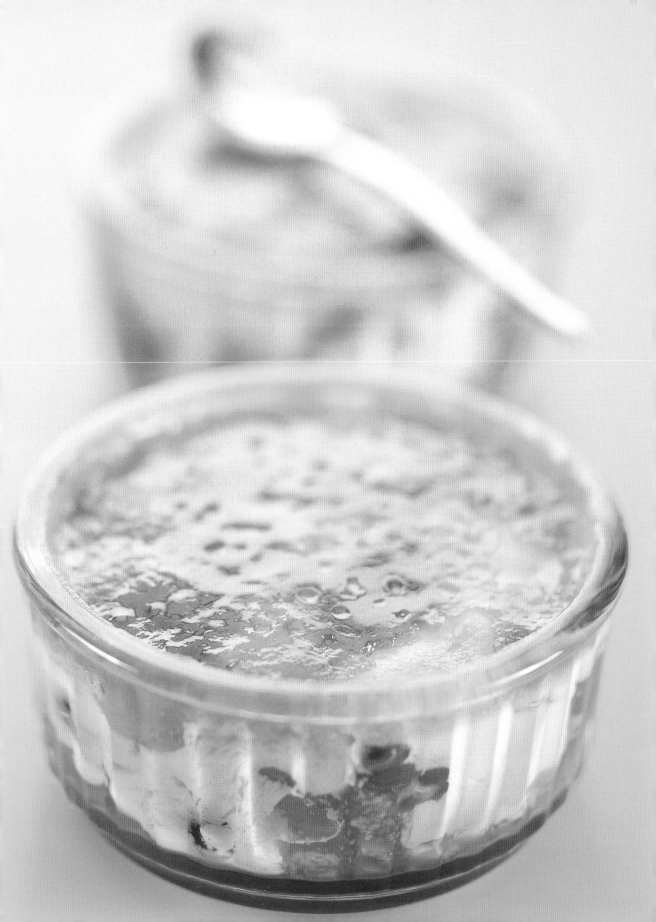

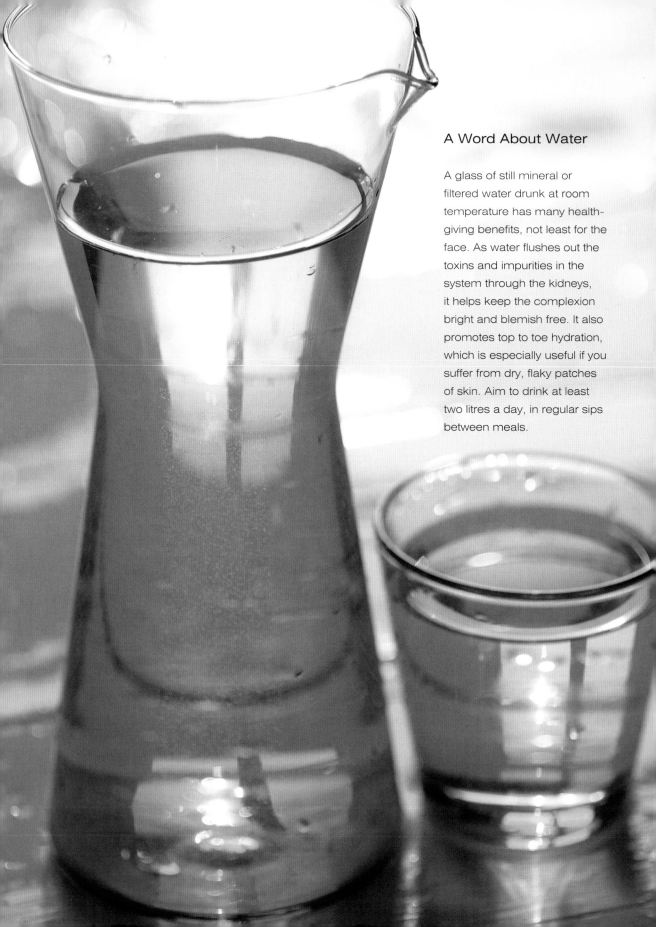

A Word About Water

A glass of still mineral or filtered water drunk at room temperature has many health-giving benefits, not least for the face. As water flushes out the toxins and impurities in the system through the kidneys, it helps keep the complexion bright and blemish free. It also promotes top to toe hydration, which is especially useful if you suffer from dry, flaky patches of skin. Aim to drink at least two litres a day, in regular sips between meals.

Skincare Basics

A simple skincare routine is the basis of a healthy complexion and the key to successful skincare is choosing the right products. It's a confusing task when you're faced with seductive advertising and an overwhelming number of products, but following a few simple rules should put you on the path to complexion perfection.

Firstly, skincare is categorized by skin type and you should match each product to the amount of oil your skin produces. If your skin is dry, you may find it looks flaky and patchy and feels tight, especially after cleansing. Normal skin is usually clear, bright and produces just enough oil to keep the skin supple. Oily complexions are often prone to blackheads and blemishes, looking shiny soon after cleansing. Combination skin is a mixture of dry and oily, with a shiny t-zone (that is the forehead, nose and chin) and drier cheeks. An increasing number of people also believe their skin is sensitive. Initially treated as a condition of very dry complexions, it is now clear that any skin type can suffer from sensitivity.

Secondly, remember that your skin is as individual as you are. Its type is not fixed for life, but will change as you get older, as your hormones fluctuate and even if you alter your environment (say by moving into an air-conditioned home or office). Every time you buy skincare products (or think that your skin type has changed), get a professional opinion from a reputable beautician before you spend anything, and shop around. Beauty counter samples are a great way of testing how your skin will generally react, but it takes around a month to see the full effects of using a new brand or regime.

If you suffer from spots or blemishes, only touch your skin with freshly washed fingers. Bacteria transfers to the skin from the hands, encouraging inflammation. Also remember that picking causes scars.

Cleanse

Removing the make-up, dirt and oil that has built up on your skin and in your pores during the day is essential for keeping it fresh and glowing. Cleansers come in many forms, from pomades, brushes and lotions to foams, gels and soaps. Some need water, others don't – base your decision on skin type and the sensation you like best. Generally speaking, drier skins will find richer creams more comforting whereas oilier skins may respond better to wash-off formulas.

Tone

Toners are a simple way to remove the last traces of grime after cleansing. Astringent toners are for oilier skins, helping to temporarily shrink pores and, if they contain matting ingredients, keep shine at bay. Containing large amounts of alcohol, astringents are not suitable if the skin is also sensitive. Toners for dry complexions usually contain soothing additives to soften the skin. If you simply want to refresh your face (and your senses), a splash of cold water will do just as well.

Moisturize

Essentially, moisturizers replenish the skin and seal in moisture after it has been cleansed and toned. Today, they are also packed with an astonishing array of ingredients aimed at particular skin types, claiming to do everything from boosting radiance to fighting ageing. Decide what your key skin concern is (wrinkles, blemishes, lacklustre tone, sun protection) and take it from there. Again, shop around and ask skincare consultants what they would recommend for you, then use a sample to test it out. Also remember that you only need to apply moisturizer on the parts of the face that feel parched – and avoid the eye area altogether. The neck should be included in your regime too, as it is also prone to the same breakouts and loss of elasticity as the rest of the face.

Skincare Extras

It may be every day or just now and again, but
sometimes the complexion needs a little extra help.

Exfoliators

The skin's top layer, the epidermis, renews itself
every twenty-eight days, but creams enhanced with
small skin-scuffing particles remove the build-up of
dead cells on the surface, keeping the complexion
bright and clear. Choose one with small round
granules that won't scratch the skin and scrub as
often as you feel your skin needs it – from once
a day to once a week.

Masks

A weekly face mask can help tackle major skincare
concerns, from deep cleansing for spot-prone
complexions to super-moisturizing for those that are
drier. They are usually left on the skin for ten to
twenty minutes, which gives the ingredients time
to really get to work.

Night creams

These are moisturizers with richer, heavier
ingredients aimed at skin that is ageing naturally or
prematurely (due to smoking or excess sun, for
example). Night creams are also a useful way to
focus on feeding your skin beneficial ingredients
because it won't need the same protection from
the elements that it needs during the day.

Eye treatments

The area of skin around the eye is extremely
delicate and needs special attention. As it is very
fine, regular moisturizer is too rich and so lighter
lotions, gels and balms are formulated to fight the
dark circles and fine lines or wrinkles that affect
that part of the face.

SOS: Know Your Skin's Enemies

Sun

The sun's UV rays damage skin on two levels.
UVA rays penetrate deep into the dermis,
causing premature ageing and skin cancer,
while the UVB rays burn the surface layers.
To help prevent sun damage, wear a sunscreen
with at least SPF15 protection during the
summer and also if you spend a long period
of time outdoors during the rest of the year.
Boosting the antioxidant quota in your diet and
using cosmetics and skincare products that
contain them, will also help skin protect itself.

Pollution

Toxins in the air form free radicals, which
contribute to the degeneration of the skin,
affecting its suppleness and plumpness.
Antioxidants will help the skin fight their effects.

Smoking

The nicotine, carbon monoxide and a host of
other nasty chemicals contained in cigarettes
not only creates free radicals but causes
a breakdown in the skin's elasticity. It also
prevents healthy blood flow to the surface of
 the skin so the complexion misses out on
oxygen and vital nutrients. The result?
A dull complexion that has more than its
share of fine lines and wrinkles.

Alcohol

Drinking dehydrates the skin, leaving it dry
and flaky. It also dilates the capillaries, making
the face look flushed and blotchy, and depletes
the body of the nutrients needed to maintain
a healthy complexion.

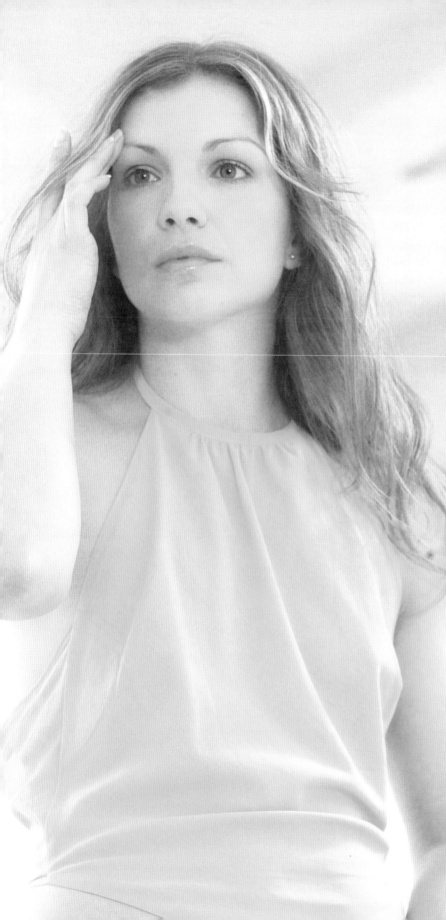

Get a Head of the Rest

Giving your beauty routine an overhaul should always include taking a closer look at how you care for your hair. On the inside, hair benefits in the same way as skin from a healthy balanced diet, rich in nutrients including iron, zinc and B vitamins. On the outside, aim for flat, smooth cuticles (the microscopic scales that coat the hair shaft) which give a glossy finish. To do this, cuticles need to be kept clean and in good condition. Ideally, you should wash your hair once a day: choose shampoo and conditioner with a formula that best suits how your hair currently feels (remember that your hair can be affected by the seasons, hormones or illness).Most of us apply too much shampoo and don't rinse for long enough, culminating in a build-up that can irritate the scalp and make hair look lank. To avoid this, ensure that you rinse hair with clean water for at least two minutes per application of shampoo. Always follow with a conditioner as it helps protect hair from pollution and the environment and keeps it supple. Wet hair is more fragile, so treat it gently: pat or blot it dry with a towel rather than rubbing, and swap harsh brushing for a gentler wide-toothed comb.

DIY Facial Massage

Massaging the face is an easy way to refresh and rejuvenate the complexion. The benefits a single five-minute session can have are immense: the circulation boost improves radiance and tone; congestion under the surface of the skin is broken down, helping to eradicate spots, blemishes and dark circles; even simply relaxing the muscles of the face will make you look more youthful.

The skin on the face is very delicate, especially around the eyes, so it's important to use lubrication, allowing the fingertips to glide easily over the surface without dragging it. Once a week, use a facial oil suited to your skin type (even oily and acne-prone skins can benefit from a gentle massage with the right oils) and indulge in this wonderful massage technique, put together by Susan Harmsworth, founder and CEO of world-leading aromatherapy company E'SPA. If you want to massage more frequently, use a pared-down version of the technique as you apply moisturizer either in the morning or at night.

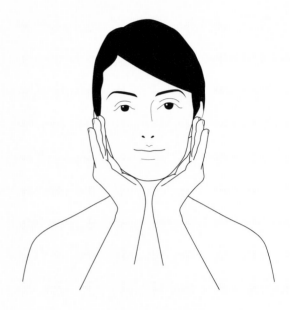

1 Dampen the skin and eye area first with a gentle toner and eye gel (E'SPA's Floral Spafresh and 24-Hour Eye Complex are ideal). Pour a few drops of facial oil into your hands and warm it by rubbing them together. Start at the base of the neck and slowly work the fingertips upwards over the face, moving out across the cheeks to the temples. With the flats of the hands, use a gentle stroking movement across the forehead from the eyebrows back to the hairline.

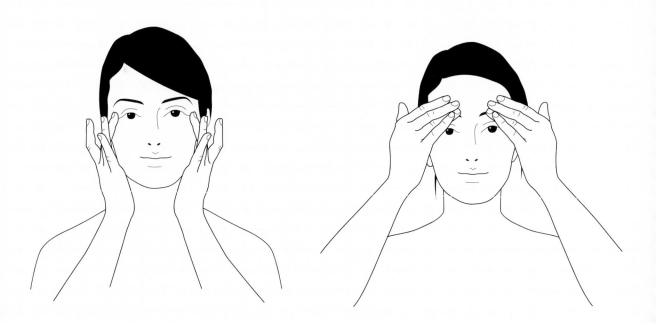

2 Circle the eyes with the ring fingers, moving in an inward direction. Then apply pressure around the eyes with the index and middle fingers, again in an inward direction. Use a gentle pumping action – press and hold, press and hold – to eliminate puffiness and dark circles.

3 A gentle lymph-drainage technique will leave the skin radiant and glowing. Using the fingertips, make light stroking movements starting from the eyebrow up into the lymph nodes along the hairline. Work down the centre of the face in lines, including under the lower lashes out to the tops of the ears. Continue until you reach just under the jawline.

Move the fingertips down to behind the base of the earlobes (this is the posterior auricle lymph node) and finish with a gentle pumping action to eliminate toxins, drain puffiness and brighten the complexion.

face and neck

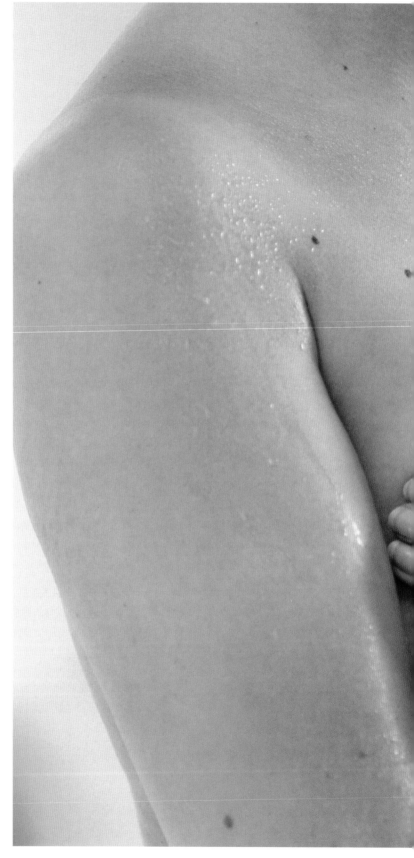

AFTER THE face, the front part of the upper body is lavished with most attention – not least because it is the next thing you see when you look down in the mirror! Toned, smooth, sculpted arms and shoulders are wonderfully attractive and once you have achieved them, easy to maintain. The décolleté too is a striking part of the body, giving definition while emphasizing femininity and, hopefully, good posture. From the collarbone to the cleavage, this area also incorporates one of the most important parts of a woman's body – her breasts.

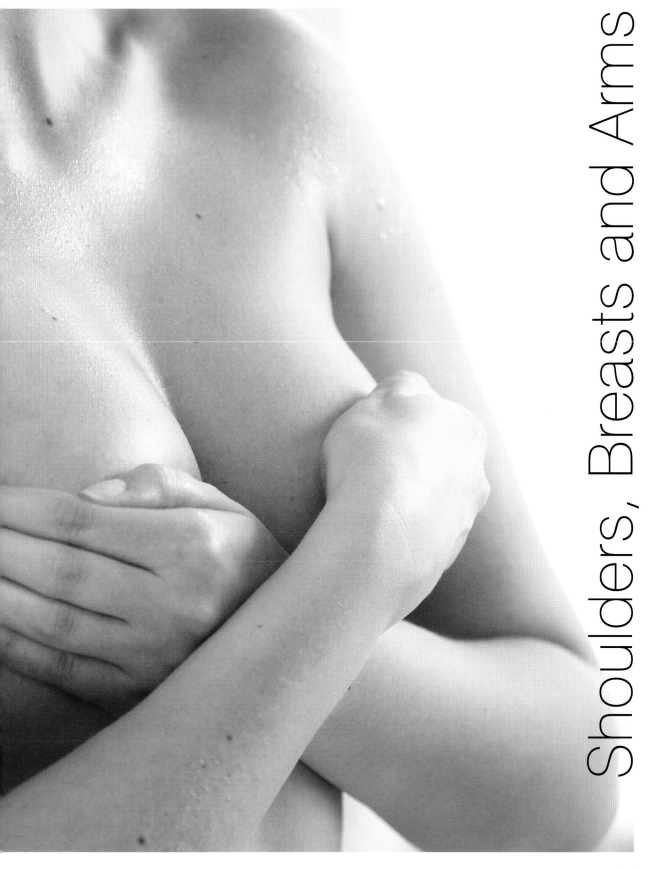

Shoulders, Breasts and Arms

Exercises for the Shoulders and Arms

The problem with modern living is that most of our activities involve rounding and closing down the upper body. We spend hours hunched over the computer, the steering wheel, the ironing board, the cooker. If we are stressed, the first place we feel it is in the neck and shoulders. We all know how good it feels to have your shoulders massaged – pure bliss – also how much better you feel when you're on holiday!

Try this: get a friend to take firm hold of both your upper arms, hunch up your shoulders but then allow your friend to take the weight of your shoulders. You can even try walking around like this, friend following and holding you. Ask your friend to release you slowly – feel the difference?

It would be great to have someone follow you all day literally taking the weight off your shoulders, but it's a little impractical! We need to learn how to release tension by ourselves. At the root of many shoulder, wrist and even hand problems is poor upper-body movement. The shoulder is one part of the body where nature has sacrificed stability for mobility – we needed a good range of movement in the shoulders to swing from the trees and reach that piece of fruit hanging from the highest branch. As a result, we rely on good muscle balance and strong ligaments to keep the shoulder joint stable.

With this in mind, Pilates exercises focus on good upper-body alignment, on releasing tension and strengthening, in particular, the muscles which set the shoulder blades down into the back, and on achieving free-flowing movement. This is what you learnt with Floating Arms (see page 25) and the Dart Stage One (see page 24). The good news is that by strengthening these muscles you are also helping to prevent unsightly folds of flesh developing around the back. Once you have established sound movement patterns then you can start toning the upper arms.

A gentle reminder though – it's no good spending hours on your Pilates exercises and then hunching back over your desk all day. Take what you have learnt in Pilates into your everyday life. Stand and sit tall, shoulders blades relaxed down into your back, chest open. You will not only feel better but you will look better too.

Scapular Squeeze (*intermediate*)

You'll feel this one working between the shoulder blades. You'll also feel the backs of your upper arms working. Your legs work too.

Aim

To strengthen the stabilizing muscles between and underneath the shoulder blades, opening the chest. To strengthen the back of the upper arms. To lengthen the spine.

Starting Position

Stand with feet parallel and hip-width apart and knees bent directly over your feet. Pivot forward on your hips as if you were skiing downhill. Look at a spot on the floor at a distance that keeps the back of your neck free from tension and the top of the head lengthening away. Too close to your feet your head will drop; too far away and you shorten the back of the neck. Take your arms behind you to the sides. The palms face upwards.

Action

1 Breathe in to prepare and lengthen up through the spine.
2 Breathe out, zip up and hollow, and slide the shoulder blades down and squeeze them and your arms together.
3 Breathe in and hold.
4 Breathe out, and release the arms.
5 Repeat five times before returning to upright. As you come upright, keep lengthening your back and head away. Return to a balanced way of standing without locking your knees.

Watchpoints

• Keep your gaze on your spot on the floor.
• Check your neck: keep it released and long.
• Think of the tailbone lengthening downwards away from the top of your head.
• Keep the knees softly bent and over your feet.

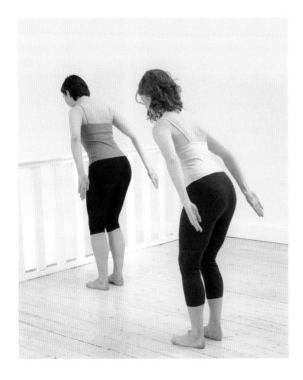
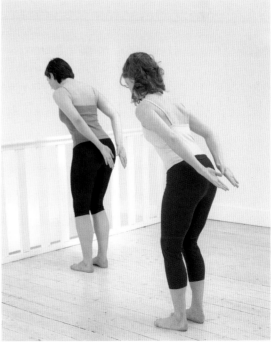

Rest Position

Aim
To lengthen and stretch out the lower back.
To make maximum use of the lungs, taking
the breath into the back.

> **Warning:** Avoid the Rest Position if you have
> knee problems as you may compress the joint.

To Get Into the Rest Position
1 Usually this exercise follows one in which you
have been lying prone (on your front), so come
up on to all fours and bring your feet together.
Your knees stay apart.

2 Slowly move your buttocks back towards your
feet. Do not raise your head or hands. Come
back to sit on your feet – not between them.
The back is rounded.

3 Rest and relax into this position. Leave the arms
extended to give you the maximum stretch. Feel
the expansion of the back of your ribcage as you
breathe deeply into it.

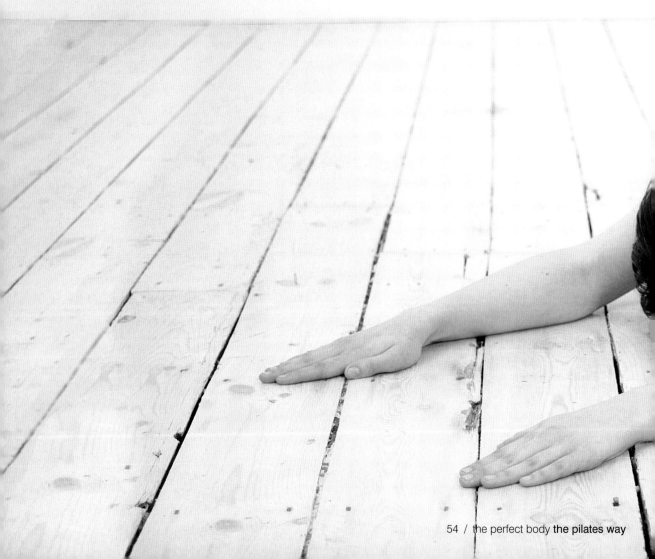

4 The further apart the knees are, the more of a stretch you will feel in your inner thighs. With the knees further apart, you can really think of your chest sinking down into the floor. You may also have the knees together which will stretch out the lumbar spine. This version may be unsuitable if you have a back injury.

5 Take ten breaths in this position.

To Come Out of the Rest Position

1 As you breathe out, zip up and hollow, and slowly unfurl.

2 Think of dropping your tailbone down and bringing your pubic bone forward.

3 Rebuild your spine vertebra by vertebra until you are upright.

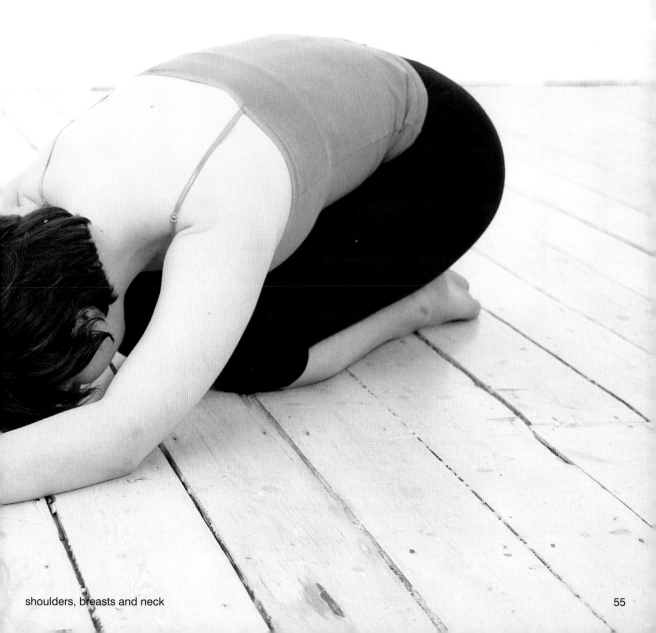

The Dart *Stage Two* (*intermediate*)

You learnt the Dart Stage One in the introduction. It is now time to work harder! There are a lot of directions in Action 2 below, so we suggest that you read them through a few times before starting the exercise.

Aim

To strengthen the mid-back muscles. You are also working the inner thighs.

Equipment

A flat pillow (optional).

Starting Position

Lie on your front. You may place a flat pillow under your forehead to allow you to breathe. Your arms are down by your sides. Your neck is long. Your legs are together, parallel, with your toes pointing.

Action

1 Breathe in to prepare and lengthen through the spine, tucking your chin in gently.
2 Breathe out, zip up and hollow, and stay zipped throughout now. Pull your shoulder blades down into your back, lengthening your fingers away from you down towards your feet. The top of your head stays lengthening away from you. Using the mid-back muscles, slowly raise the upper body a few centimetres from the floor. Keep looking straight down. Do not tip your head back. Meanwhile, squeeze your inner thighs together but keep your feet on the floor.
3 Breathe in and feel the length of your body from the tips of your toes to the top of your head.
4 Breathe out, still zipped, and slowly lower.
5 Repeat up to six times.

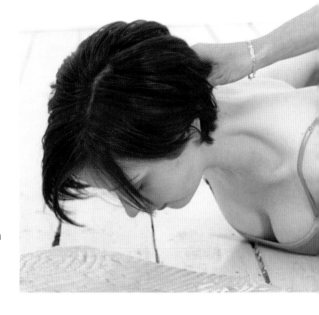

This exercise should be followed by the Rest Position on page 54.

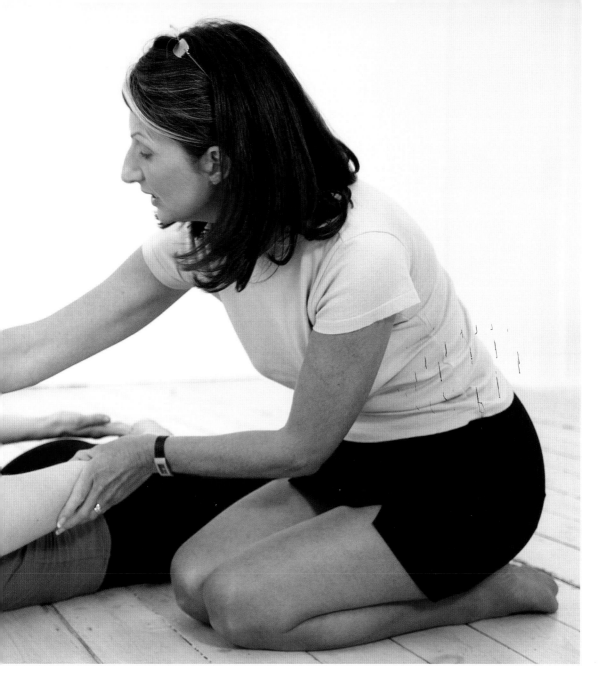

Watchpoints

- Keep hollowing the lower abdominals.
- Do not strain the neck, it should feel released as your shoulders engage down into your back. Think of a swan's neck growing out between its wings.
- Remember to keep your feet on the floor.
- Please stop if you feel at all uncomfortable in the low back.

This exercise can also be done with the feet hip-width apart and the thigh and buttock muscles relaxed.

shoulders, breasts and neck

Up and Over (*intermediate*)

A great exercise for opening the upper body and getting a good range of movement in the shoulders.

Aim
To learn correct upper-body use. To open the upper body, gently stretching the front of the chest.

Equipment
A long scarf or a stretchband.

Starting Position
Stand correctly (see page 6), lengthening through the spine. Hold the scarf lightly in front of you with both hands, about one metre apart.

Action
1 Breathe in wide and full to prepare.
2 Breathe out and zip up and hollow. Stay zipped now, as you raise the scarf, allowing the movement of the hands to lead the arms and shoulders. Try to keep the upper shoulders relaxed – don't let them hike up around your ears. Think of the shoulder blades dropping down as the arms rise. Make the movement initiate from your shoulder blades.
3 Breathe in and, keeping the arms straight but not locked, take the scarf behind you in a wide arc.
4 Breathe in as you slowly raise the scarf from behind, and breathe out as you slowly bring it back down in front.

Watchpoints
- As you raise your arms try to keep good alignment throughout the body; do not tilt the upper body backwards.
- Keep zipped, please.
- If you have to bend an elbow or duck your head as the scarf moves behind you, try holding it wider. If it is still difficult you are not ready for this so keep practising the other shoulder exercises until you are more flexible.

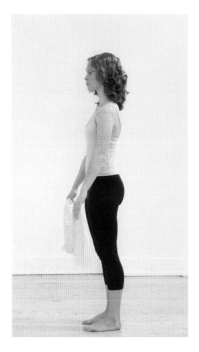
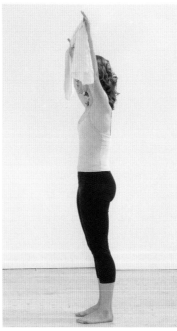
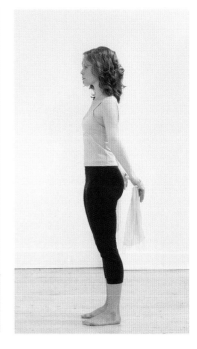

Standing Tarzan (*beginners*)

A fun exercise in the standing-weights series. It targets the upper-arm muscles.

Aim
To strengthen the biceps.

Equipment
Light hand-held weights up to 1 kilo each weight.

Starting Position
Stand correctly (see page 6). Once you are comfortable with the movement you can use the weights. Hold your arms out to the sides, shoulder blades down into your back, neck released. Have the arms straight but not locked.

Action
1 Breathe in wide and full, and lengthen up through the spine.
2 Breathe out and zip up and hollow. Stay gently zipped and slowly curl your arms in towards your head, hingeing from the elbows.
3 Breathe in and slowly straighten the arm again.
4 Repeat eight times.

Watchpoints
- Keep the upper arm quite still.
- As you straighten the arms think of lengthening away.

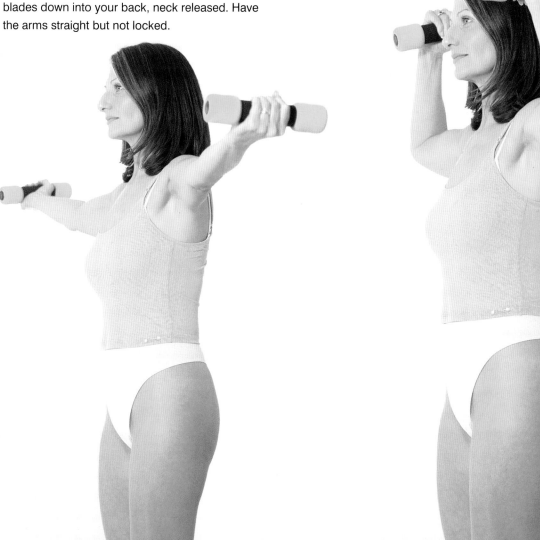
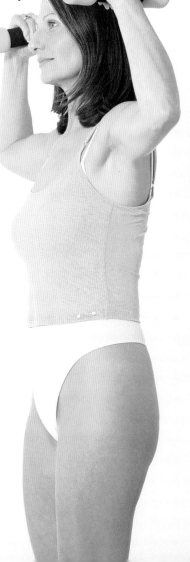

Standing Backstroke
(beginners without weights, intermediate with weights)

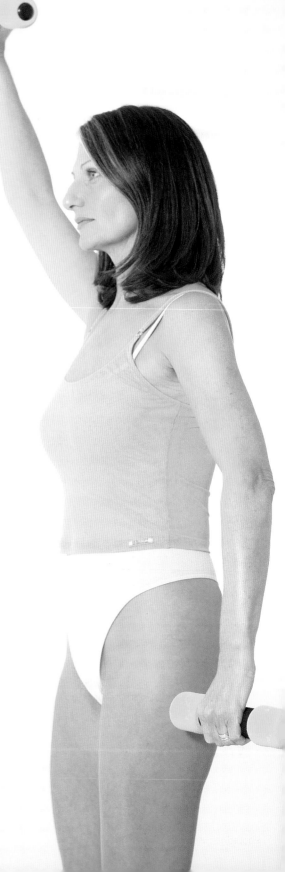

The following set of exercises is designed to teach you good upper-body mechanics and also tones the arms and the shoulders. Yo-yo dieting often leaves the upper arms flabby with excess skin. You have to work hard to target this area. What we are aiming for is well-defined arms, nicely sculpted, but without looking bulky and masculine. Practise first without weights and then try with light hand-held weights of about 500 grams each weight. This is great for sculpting the arms and also for building bone density, so it is a good exercise for the prevention and treatment of osteoporosis.

Aim
To tone the arms and shoulders.

Equipment
Light weights.

Starting Position
Stand correctly (see page 6), with your arms relaxed down by your sides, palms facing backwards.

Action
1 Breathe in wide and full and lengthen through the top of your head.
2 Breathe out and zip up and hollow. Stay zipped now, and raise your right arm above your head, remembering everything you learnt in Floating Arms (see page 25). Shoulder blades dropping, neck released.

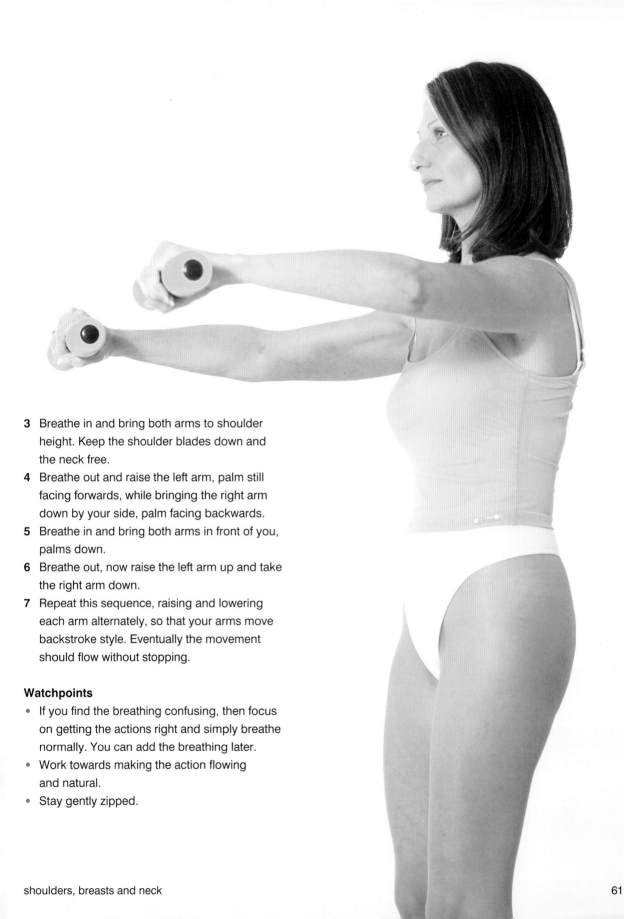

3 Breathe in and bring both arms to shoulder
  height. Keep the shoulder blades down and
  the neck free.
4 Breathe out and raise the left arm, palm still
  facing forwards, while bringing the right arm
  down by your side, palm facing backwards.
5 Breathe in and bring both arms in front of you,
  palms down.
6 Breathe out, now raise the left arm up and take
  the right arm down.
7 Repeat this sequence, raising and lowering
  each arm alternately, so that your arms move
  backstroke style. Eventually the movement
  should flow without stopping.

Watchpoints

- If you find the breathing confusing, then focus
  on getting the actions right and simply breathe
  normally. You can add the breathing later.
- Work towards making the action flowing
  and natural.
- Stay gently zipped.

shoulders, breasts and neck

Mermaid (*intermediate*)

A lovely exercise for stretching out your waist and strengthening the upper body.

Starting Position

Sit on the floor facing forwards with both knees bent towards your right-hand side. Have the knees a comfortable distance away from your body in a line with each other. Your weight will be on your left hip. Lightly clasp the front of your right shin with your right hand. Even though you are sitting at an angle, keep lengthening up through the spine.

Action

1 Breathe in wide and lengthen up through the spine.

2 Breathe out and zip up and hollow. Stay zipped now and float your left arm up, dropping the shoulder blade down into your back, your palm faces inward.

3 Breathe in wide and full, lengthening up, up up.

4 Breathe out, and reach the left arm across to the right aiming for the top corner of the room. Reach through the fingertips, feel the stretch between your ribs and your hips along the left side.

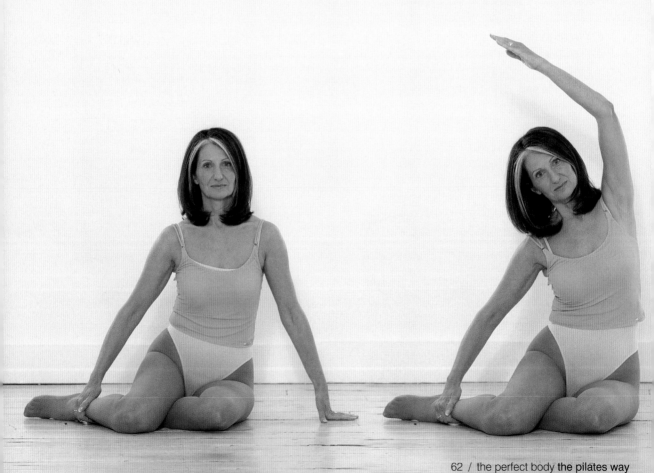

5 Breathe in wide and come back to centre.

6 Breathe out and lower the left arm to the floor, coming on to the elbow and forearm if you can, and raise the right arm to reach across to the left, palm facing away from you. Enjoy the stretch along your right side. Keep your right hip down to increase the stretch.

7 Breathe in and push up on the left elbow and forearm to return to the starting position.

8 Use the momentum of coming up to carry you through on the out breath, stretching to the right once again.

9 Repeat five times this side and then repeat five times on the other side.

Watchpoints

- Keep your movement slow and flowing, a bit like a reed bending in the wind.
- Try to stretch directly to each side in the same plane, without tilting forward or back.

> **Warning:** take advice if you have back or sacroiliac problems.

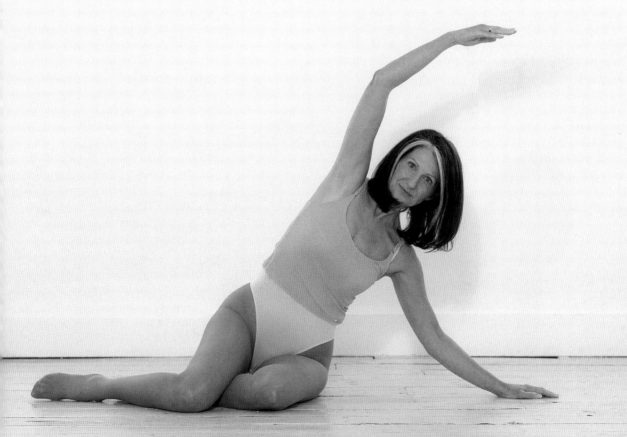

Side Bends (*advanced*)

Aim
To improve overall strength. Think long and strong.

> **Warning:** avoid this exercise if you have shoulder, arm or neck problems.

Starting Position
Lie in a straight line on your right side with your legs stretched out. Put your right forearm on the floor at right angles to your body. Bend your right elbow so that your head and upper body are propped up on your forearm. Your left hand rests softly on the floor in front of you. Take your left leg and place it over and in front of the right leg. Keep your left foot close to the ankle of the right, with your left foot pointing forward and the sole flat on the mat.

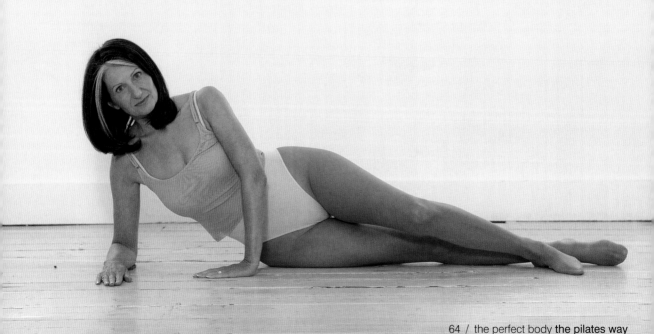

Action

1 Breathe in wide and full to prepare and lengthen through the spine.

2 Breathe out and zip up and hollow. Stay zipped now and lift your left hip up to the ceiling by pushing into your left foot. At the same time float the left arm up and over your head to reach across to the top corner of the room. Squeeze your inner thighs together.

3 Breathe out and slowly lower the whole body to the mat, circling the left arm back down.

4 Repeat up to five times on each side.

Watchpoints

- When you have lifted your body from the mat try to keep your pelvis and spine in neutral. Do not let the pelvis roll forward.
- It helps to imagine a large thick strap wrapped around your hips and lifting you up towards the ceiling.
- Try not to push into the shoulders and arms, they will be working but your weight should be on the front foot.
- Remember to think long and strong.

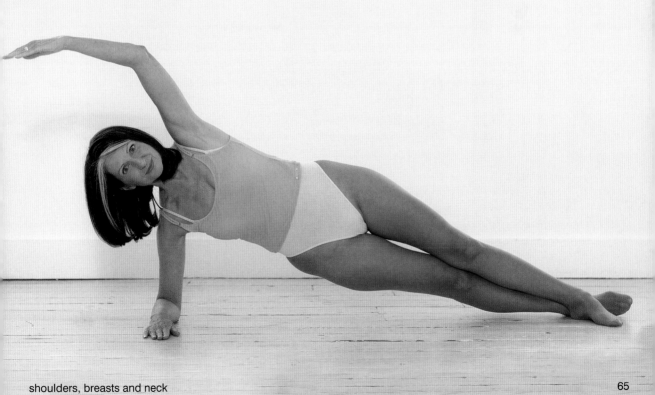

shoulders, breasts and neck

The Perfect Décolleté

Be it in a bikini or a low-cut evening dress, the décolleté is an area that can be used to emphasize the shape and definition of the upper body. While you work on sculpting the area with the Pilates exercises on the previous pages, combine these priming tips into your daily beauty routine. Then, when you are ready to reveal all, make the most of your new appearance with a light dusting of shade or shimmer.

Prime

As the arms and chest are often exposed during summer, they are prone to showing signs of sun damage. Thankfully, with regular attention the skin will quickly improve in texture, tone and clarity. Follow these simple steps:

- If you are spending any length of time outdoors, help prevent premature fine lines and wrinkles, age spots and roughened texture by applying a sunscreen to your bare arms and chest. Choose a minimum of SPF15 and increase the factor during high summer or when you are travelling to hotter climates.
- When you exfoliate in the bath or shower, remember to include the arms, bust and chest, as they are prone to blocked pores and sluggish circulation (for the best exfoliators, read Skin Essentials on page 92).
- A daily application of bust treatment will help firm the fine skin there, helping to prevent sagging, stretch marks and wrinkles in the future. Those by Clarins, Yves Saint Laurent and Shu Uemura are favourites all over the world.

Each of these easy make-up tricks will give the décolleté a different look. Choose the effect to match your outfit and your invitation!

Bronzing

A light application of wear-off self-tan or wash-off bronzing gel is ideal for a golden glow. As well as giving a fresh, healthy appearance, the colour will help to hide any age spots or blemishes. Make sure you leave enough time for it to dry thoroughly after application to avoid streaks and stained clothes.

Shading

For sultry definition, choose a taupe or honey-toned shading powder that will add a mixture of shadows and light to the chest. Use a large blusher or powder brush and gently sweep the colour in a soft V-shape between the breasts (and down the side if it is exposed) to create contours. Gradually building the powder up in stages rather than overdoing it on the first sweep is a foolproof way to apply it evenly.

Shimmering

Create pretty highlights with pearlized or iridescent colour blended along the collarbone, across the shoulders and even down the back. There are a multitude of textures to choose from – cream, gel, stick, powder – each with a different depth and staying power, so play around and experiment! From gold to glittery, these highlighters are the perfect way to turn a plain outfit into a stunning ensemble.

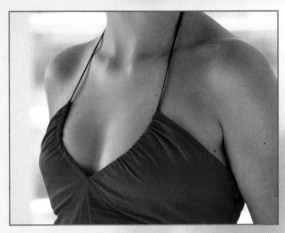

Bronzing

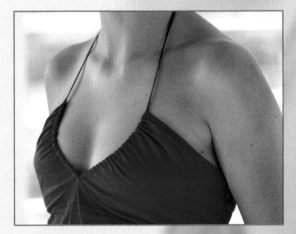

Shading

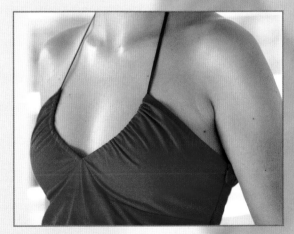

Shimmering

Breast Health

With the number of women suffering from breast cancer increasing each year, it is essential that women take an active role in the health of their breasts. The sections that follow will give you an idea of the factors you need to be aware of and simple suggestions which you can adopt into your lifestyle, but if you do have any concerns, contact your doctor, health specialist or national breast cancer association for further information and advice.

Fit Right

Many department stores now offer a professional bra-fitting service in their lingerie departments and with good reason – an estimated nine out of ten women buy underwear that is the wrong size. While there is still some discussion as to how much wearing a bra contributes to the health of the breasts, one thing is for certain – a badly fitting bra will not do them any good. The breasts are supported not by muscles but by ligaments that stretch naturally with age, causing sagging and drooping.

A well-fitted bra helps prevent this process as well as offering comfort and giving the bust a good shape. If your bra is too tight, it can cause pain in the back, neck and shoulders, poor posture and even breathing difficulties. If your bra is too loose, it will not provide the breasts with enough support.

Have your bra size checked regularly and when you start or finish taking the contraceptive pill, become pregnant or gain or lose a significant amount of weight.

DIY Breast Check

A monthly breast examination should be a crucial part of every woman's calendar. Early detection of breast cancer certainly saves lives, and if you do see or feel any irregularities, make an appointment with your doctor immediately. As you examine yourself, look for:

- Continual pain in any part of the breast.
- Unusual changes in the shape or size of either breast.
- One breast becoming lower and changing shape.
- Any lumps or thickening within the breast or under the arm.
- A rash or change of skin colour around either nipple.
- A change in the shape or position of either nipple.
- Discharge from one or both nipples.

It is normal for the breasts to change shape and size during your menstrual cycle as they are controlled by your hormones, so examine them at the same time each month, just after the end of your period. If you no longer have periods, stick to the same date each month.

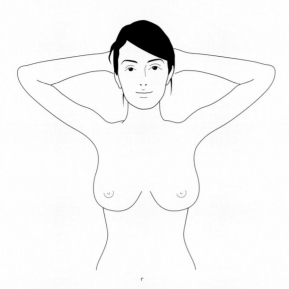

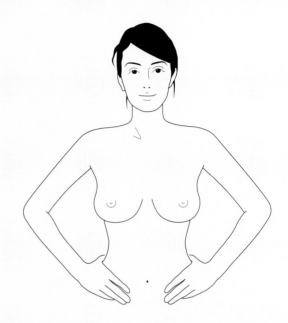

Begin by looking at the shape, size and positioning of your breasts in the mirror. Stand straight on and turn to each side, first with your hands down and then above your head.

Place your hands on your hips and tip your body forwards and backwards, always watching for any unusual changes.

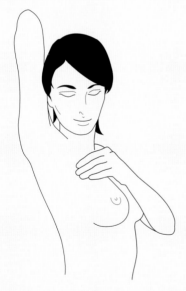

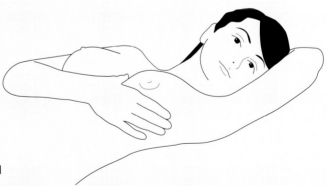

Using the first two fingers of the opposite hand, feel each breast in turn. Apply a firm pressure with the fingertips and move around the entire breast with small circular motions. Make sure you cover the entire breast – from the armpit, over the top of the breast, then across and underneath it. You should also feel around the collarbone for any swelling.

Finish by lying down and repeating this sequence.

Diet and Breast Health

The role of diet in the prevention of cancer has been increasingly examined in the past few years, sparking great debate among medical and nutrition experts. Some studies suggest that a high-fat diet, particularly one that is rich in saturated fats, may increase the risk of breast cancer, while a diet rich in fruit and vegetables can reduce this risk. Other factors that may increase your susceptibility are a high intake of alcohol and meat.

Recent research suggests that a diet rich in soya may help protect against breast cancer. Soya beans and products made from them, such as tofu and soya milk, are packed full of compounds called isoflavones. Isoflavones have a similar structure to the hormone oestrogen and can bind to oestrogen receptor sites throughout the body, mimicking its natural effect. In doing so, they are thought to reduce the rate at which cells divide, lowering the likelihood of breast cancer cells developing. There is also some evidence to suggest that a diet packed with carotenoid compounds (found in highly coloured fruit and vegetables such as carrots, red, yellow and orange peppers, pumpkin and apricots) may also reduce the risk.

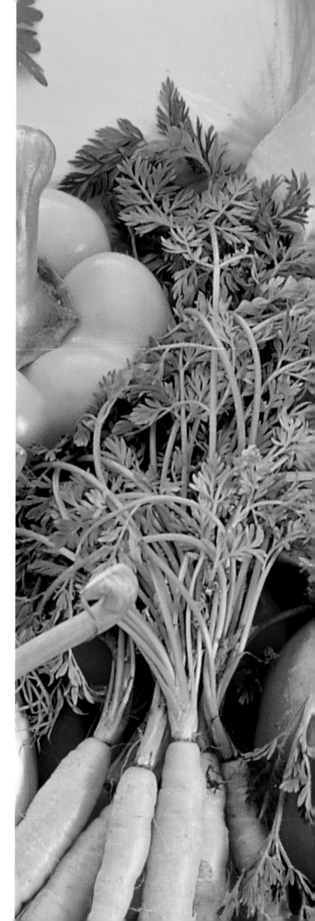

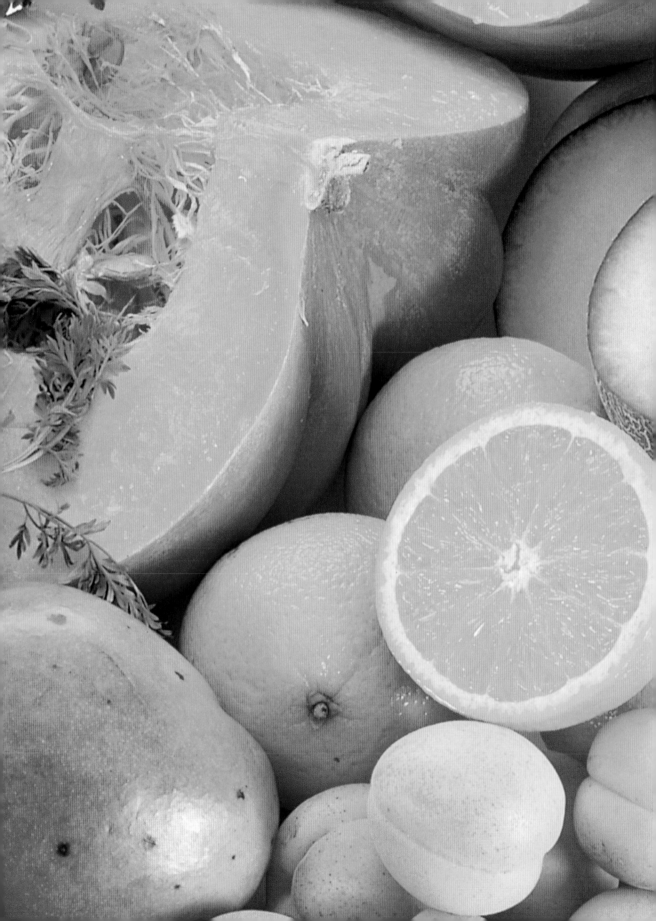

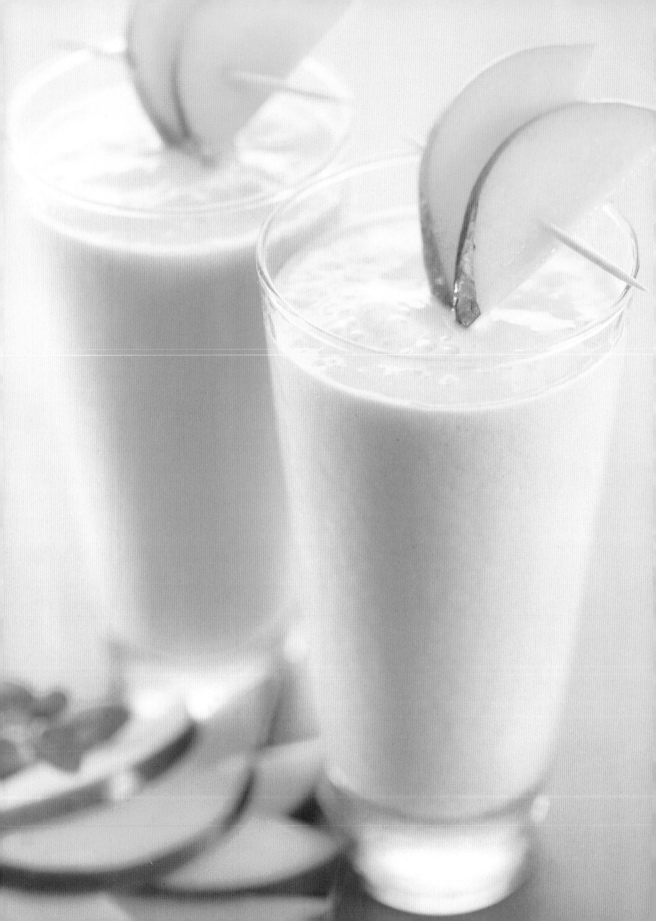

Mango Smoothie

Preparation time: **5 minutes,**
Cooking time: **nil**
Serves: **1**

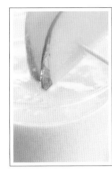

1 large ripe mango, peeled and chopped
200ml soya milk
150ml soya yoghurt

Put the mango with the other ingredients in a blender
and purée until smooth.

Add a couple of ice cubes and drink immediately.

Tofu Kebabs with Indonesian Salad

Preparation time: **15 minutes**
Cooking time: **10 minutes**
Serves: **4**

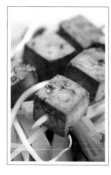

for the tofu kebabs:

1 clove garlic, finely chopped

3 tbsp dark soy sauce

1 tsp dark muscovado sugar

250g firm tofu, cut into
     1cm pieces

8 bamboo skewers

for the satay sauce:

1 tbsp vegetable oil

1 garlic clove, crushed or
     finely chopped

2 tsp chilli powder

225g crunchy peanut butter

1 tbsp dark muscovado sugar

finely grated zest of 1 large
     lemon

300ml water

for the salad:

400g white cabbage, cut into
     narrow strips

4 carrots, cut into thick julienne

340g beansprouts

340g sugar snap peas, trimmed

175g broccoli florets, cut small

Mix together the garlic, soy sauce and sugar. Toss the tofu in the mixture. Cover and leave to marinate for at least an hour.

Soak 8 bamboo skewers in cold water for 30 minutes.

To make the satay sauce, heat the oil in a saucepan and add the garlic and chilli powder. Stir for 1–2 minutes. Add the peanut butter, sugar, lemon zest and water. Bring to a simmer and cook for 4–5 minutes until the sauce thickens.

To make the salad, blanch all the vegetables in boiling water for about 2–3 minutes so that they do not lose their crunchiness. Drain well.

Preheat the grill to high. Thread the tofu onto the skewers and cook for 3–4 minutes on each side, turning occasionally, until browned.

Serve two skewers per person on a bed of vegetables, with the satay sauce spooned on top.

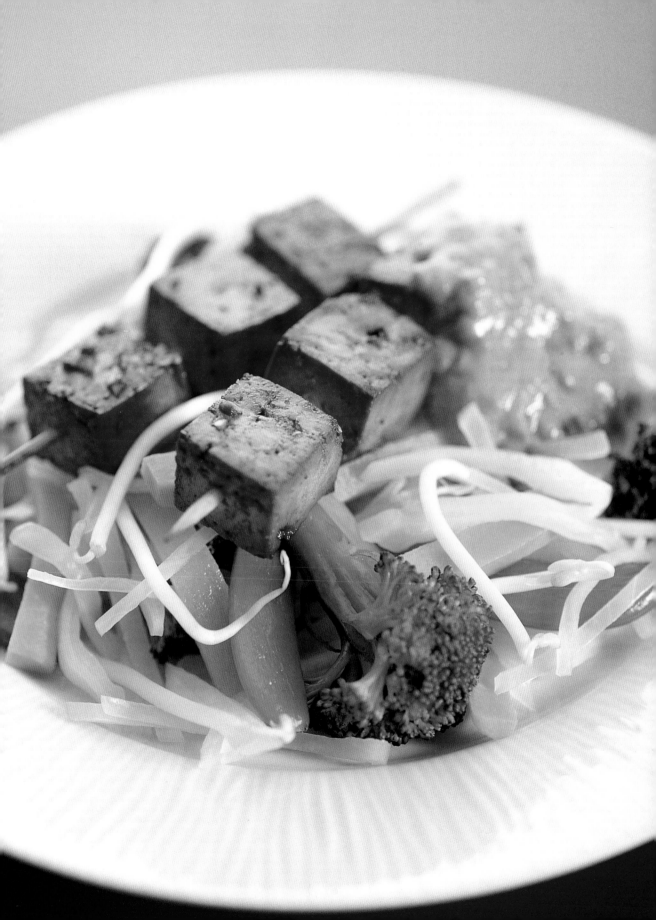

THE BACK is an underestimated part of the body. It includes the spine, which plays a crucial role in holding you upright and creating good posture. For this reason, keeping it strong and healthy with a balanced programme of exercises is essential. A toned and sculpted back is also sensual and beautiful to look at, so whether you're in need of a blemish-clearing mask or a muscle-easing back rub, it's worth enlisting the help of a friend to reach those parts that you can't reach yourself.

It's a pity that good posture has become so unfashionable over the last few decades because your grandmother knew what she was talking about when she told you to stop slouching and stand up straight! The benefits of good posture are endless. You can breathe better (try hunching and then breathing wide and full – it's impossible because the ribcage has collapsed). You will digest your food better. You will lessen·wear and tear on all your joints, thus reducing the likelihood of developing everything from osteoarthritis to repetitive strain injuries. There'll be no dowager's hump as you grow older because you will retain a youthful spine.

If we haven't convinced you yet, just think about how you really look when you slouch.

Have you ever caught a sideways glimpse of yourself in a mirror when you're out and been shocked? Doubtless you reacted automatically by standing up straighter because in so doing, you instantly looked taller, slimmer and younger. When you hunch, your breasts look saggy and low slung, your waist disappears and your stomach sticks out – not a good look.

Pilates is essentially a postural re-education technique. Every exercise in this book will take you one step closer to good posture. But there's no point practising Pilates and then forgetting everything you have learnt when you are at work or at home. To avoid undoing all the good you have done, make Pilates a part of every aspect of your life. When you are walking down the street, imagine that a balloon is attached to the top of your head and you will float along the pavement. Gently zip up and hollow as you wait for the bus. As you queue in traffic think of lengthening up through the spine, relaxing the shoulder blades down into your back, softening your breastbone, opening your elbows, releasing your jaw and neck – feel the stresses of city driving melt away.

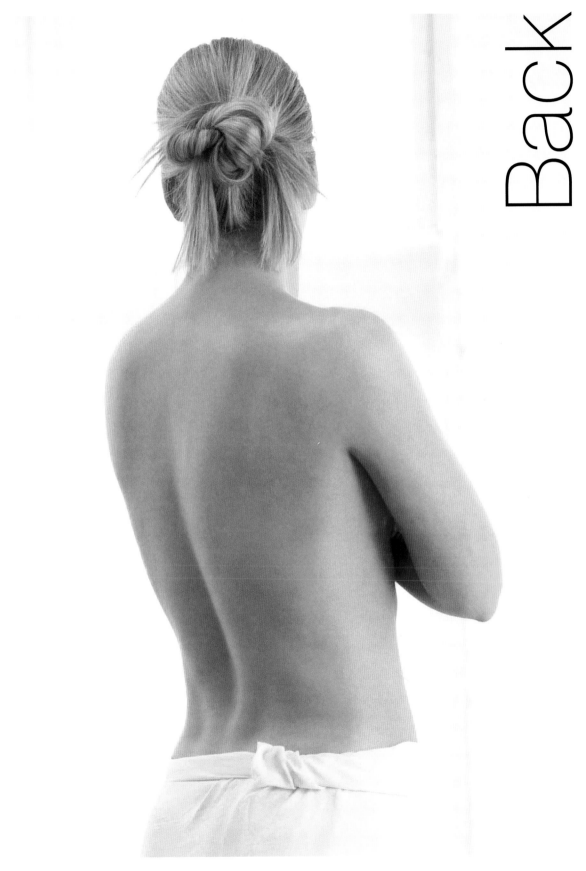

Exercises for the Back

Joseph Pilates was always reminding his clients that you are only as old as your spine. Any balanced fitness programme must include all the movements that the spine can perform – flexion (forward bending), extension (backward bending), rotation (twisting) and lateral flexion (side bending). In a healthy spine, each vertebra moves independently of its neighbour – no sections are locked or jammed, a bit like a string of pearls. The vertebrae float on the discs. You can imagine these discs being like rubber balls between the bony vertebrae, cushioning and supporting the bones.

In earthquake-prone countries, buildings are often built on rubber cylinders (discs) alternating with metal cylinders (vertebrae) to help absorb the shock of tremors, and the spine is built in a similar way to absorb shock. In Pilates, we try to promote mobility and segmental control by saying that every time you peel the spine from the mat or replace the spine on the mat, do so vertebra by vertebra, bone by bone, lengthening all the time.

The following exercises will keep your spine supple and strong.

Spine Curls with Pillow (*beginners*)

A wonderful exercise for the spine. Squeezing the pillow will also target those inner thighs and make the buttocks work as well. To make this exercise more challenging perform it with the arms behind you, wide and open, on the mat. You should be able to do this without the ribs flaring or the upper back arching.

Aim
To learn how to wheel the spine, vertebra by vertebra, achieving synchronous segmental control. To work the adductors, the inner thigh muscles.

Equipment
A plump pillow.

Starting Position

Lie in the Relaxation Position (see page 14), but have your arms down by your sides and your feet together, perfectly lined up, about thirty centimetres away from your buttocks. Place the pillow between your knees. Your arms are relaxed down by your sides, palms down.

Action

1 Breathe in to prepare.
2 Breathe out and zip up and hollow. Squeeze the pillow between the knees and curl the tailbone off the floor just a little.
3 Breathe in and then breathe out, zip up and hollow, and slowly curl back down lengthening out the spine.
4 Breathe out, zip up and hollow and peel a little more of the spine off the floor.
5 Breathe in and then breathe out and, zip up and hollow as you place the spine back down, bone by bone.
6 Continue to curl more of the spine off the floor. Each time you go up on the exhalation. Inhale while you are raised and then exhale as you wheel the spine, vertebra by vertebra, back down on the floor. Aim to lengthen the spine as you wheel back down. The deep abdominals and pelvic floor stay engaged throughout and you keep squeezing the pillow.

Watchpoints

- You must not arch the back. Keep in your mind the image of a whippet who has just been scolded, his tail (your tailbone) curled between his legs.
- Keep the weight even on both feet and try not to let the feet roll in or out.
- Keep your neck long and soft.

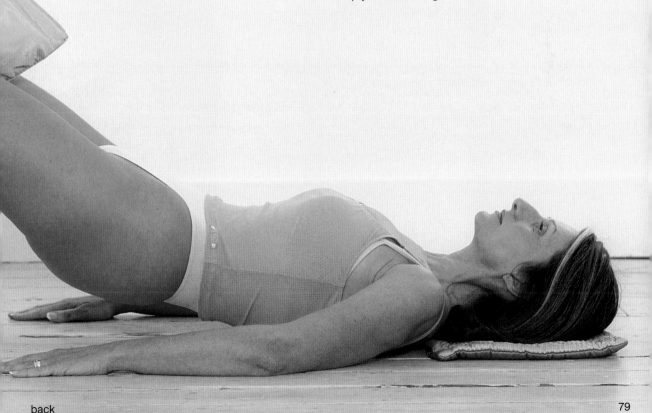

Side Reach Against the Wall (*beginners*)

This takes the spine into lateral flexion. It stretches and works the waist too. By doing the exercise against a wall you can better judge your alignment. But, of course, you can also do this exercise freestanding.

Aim
To stretch the sides of the trunk and learn good lateral flexion of the spine.

Starting Position
Stand with your back to a wall and your feet a few centimetres away from it. Have them just wider than shoulder-width apart and facing forward. Notice where your body touches the wall. Do not tip your head back; check that your pelvis is in neutral. Your hands are resting on the outsides of your thighs. You are going to keep the non-working arm in contact with the outside of the thigh throughout the stretch.

Action
1 Breathe in wide and full to prepare and lengthen through the spine.
2 Breathe out and zip up and hollow. Stay zipped throughout, and slowly raise one arm up to the side and above your head trying to keep it in contact with the wall, but do not force it.

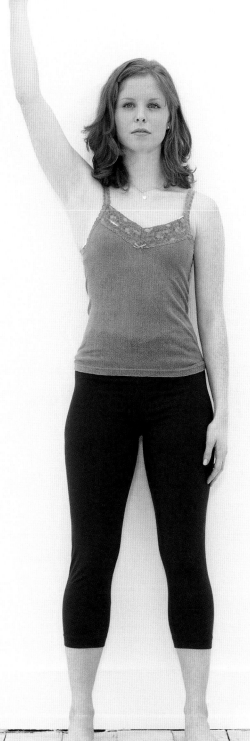

3 Breathe in wide and just check that your shoulder blade is still connected down into your back and that there is a large gap between your ear and your shoulder. Lengthen up through the top of your head.
4 Breathe out, still zipped, and lift up out of your waist to reach towards the corner of the ceiling. Keep your head in a line with your spine (face forward still) and do not move away from the wall.
5 Breathe in and slowly return to the centre.
6 Breathe out and lower the arm along the wall.
7 Repeat five times to each side.

Watchpoints

* Keep noting where your body is touching the wall.
* Keep your pelvis central and do not allow it to shift to one side.
* Keep both feet firmly on the floor.
* Try to open out from the waist, moving the ribcage away from the hips rather than just reaching through the arm.

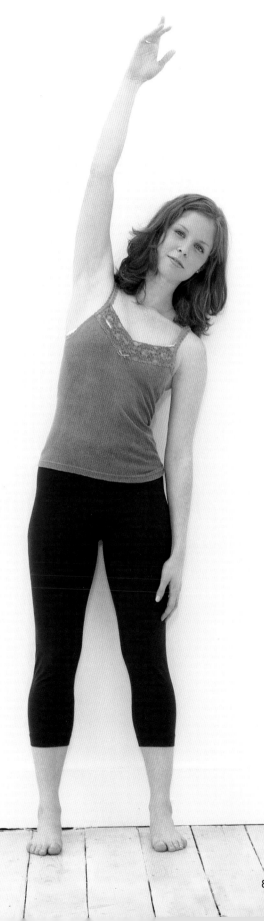

Roll Downs (*intermediate*)

A core exercise in any Pilates programme. It can be used as a warm up or a wind down. It combines stabilizing work with the wonderful wheeling motion of the spine. As you roll back up think of rebuilding the spinal column, stacking each vertebra one on top of the other to lengthen out the spine.

For the advanced version
Try holding light weights – 500 grams each weight – as you do this, it helps relax the shoulders.

Aim
To release tension in the spine, the shoulders and the upper body. To mobilize the spine, creating flexibility and strength and achieving segmental control. To teach the correct way of stabilizing the abdominals when bending.

Starting Position
Stand with your feet hip-width apart and parallel, and your weight evenly balanced on both feet. Check that you are not rolling your feet in or out. Soften your knees. Find your neutral pelvis position but keep the tailbone lengthening down.

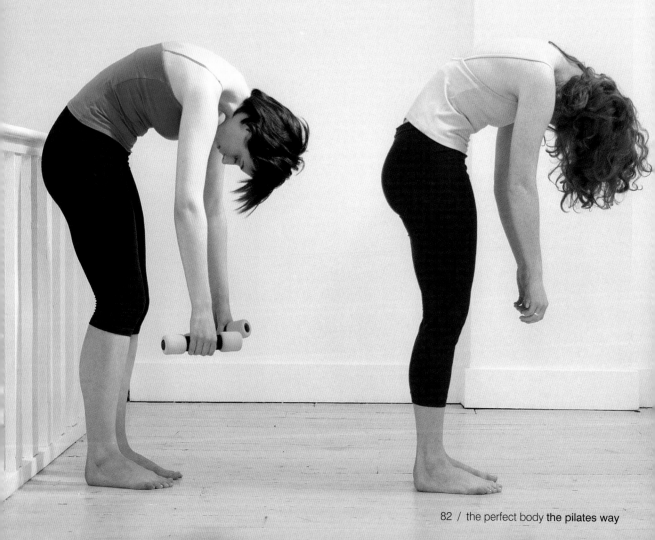

Action

1 Breathe in to prepare and lengthen up through the spine. Release the head and the neck.
2 Breathe out, zip up and hollow and drop your chin onto your chest and allow the weight of your head to make you slowly roll forward, head released, arms hanging, centre strong, knees soft.
3 Breathe in as you hang, really let your head and arms hang.
4 Breathe out, firmly zipped, as you drop your tailbone down, directing your pubic bone forward, and rotate your pelvis backwards as you slowly come up to standing tall, rolling through the spine bone by bone.
5 Repeat six times.

Watchpoints

• You may like to take an extra breath during the exercise. This is fine but please try to breathe out as you move the spine.
• Make sure that you go down centrally. Do not sway over to one side. When you are down, check where your hands are in relation to your feet.
• Do not roll the feet in or out. Keep the weight evenly balanced and try not to lean forwards on to the front of your feet or backwards on to the heels.

> **Warning:** take advice if you have a back problem, especially if it is disc related.

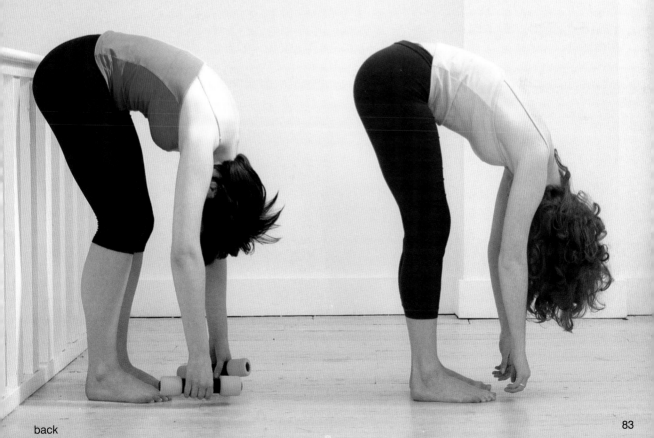

back

The Cat (*beginners*)

A feel-good exercise that unknots the spine
while teaching you good alignment.

Aim
To mobilize the spine and learn correct alignment.

Starting Position
Kneel on all fours with your hands placed directly
beneath your shoulders, the fingers facing forwards.
Your knees should be in line with your hips, the
lower leg straight. Look straight down at the floor so
that the back of your neck is long. Find the natural
neutral curve in your spine. Think of a pool of
water in the small of your back. Keep lengthening
the top of your head away from your tailbone.
Your shoulder blades should be down into your
back. Do not be tempted to lock your elbows.
Keep your weight on the whole of the hand, not
just the heels.

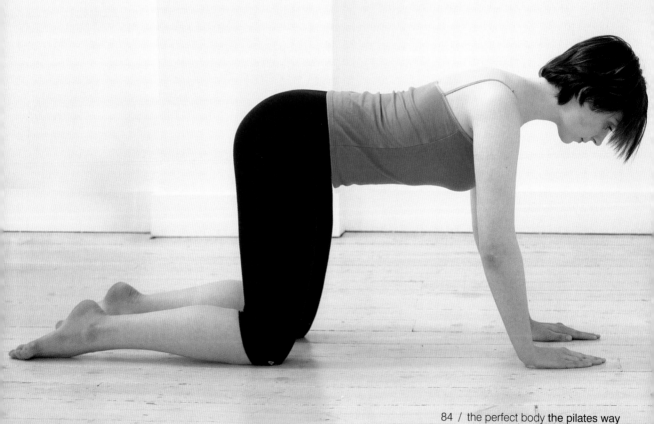

Action

1 Breathe in wide and full to prepare and lengthen through the spine.

2 Breathe out and zip up and hollow. Stay zipped throughout and, starting with the base of the spine, begin to curl your tailbone under – a bit like you did for Spine Curls on page 78. Work your way up the back, rounding it, but keeping it open and wide. Your chin will end up tucked in toward your chest; neck and head released. Imagine a hook pulling you up from the back of the waist to the ceiling.

3 Breathe in wide, checking that your elbows haven't locked.

4 Breathe out, and slowly uncurl the spine starting again from the base, sticking your tailbone out, mobilizing vertebra by vertebra, sliding the shoulder blades down into your back, until you have returned to neutral. Please do not over-dip the low back or lift the head back. Feel the length of the spine.

5 Repeat five times.

Watchpoints

- Keep the weight even on both hands.
- If your wrists tire, stop for a short break, then start again. Eventually they will strengthen. Or you can try placing folded towels under the heel of the hands to reduce the angle at the wrist.
- Focus on moving the spine bone by bone.
- Remember not to lock your elbows.

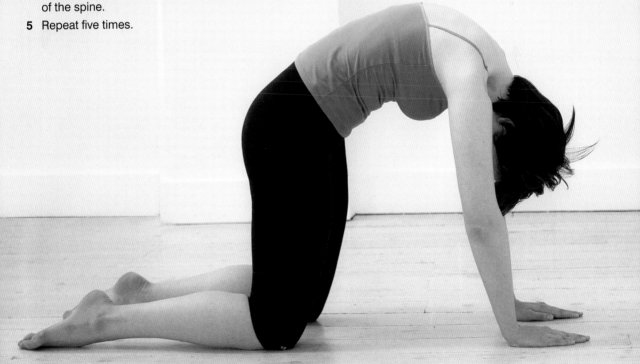

Bow and Arrow (*beginners*)

There are many Pilates exercises that encourage rotation of the spine, for example Hip Rolls on pages 99–100. This is a favourite, however, as it really opens the upper body and teaches you to turn while lengthening.

Starting Position

Sit tall with your legs bent in front of you. If you have the flexibility, you should stretch your legs out straight. Make sure that you are sitting on your sitting bones (ischia). Hold your arms out in front of you, at shoulder height, palms facing down. Your shoulder blades are down into your back and your neck is released.

Action

1 Breathe in wide and full and lengthen through the spine.
2 Breathe out, zip up and hollow and stay zipped throughout now.
3 Breathe in and fold your left hand in towards your chest; the elbow stays up in a line with the shoulder.
4 Still on the in breath, turn the upper body, unfolding the arm so it straightens out behind you. Your head follows the arm but stays in a line with your spine. Your upper body is now open.
5 Breathe out, and bring the arm back to the front in a wide circle.

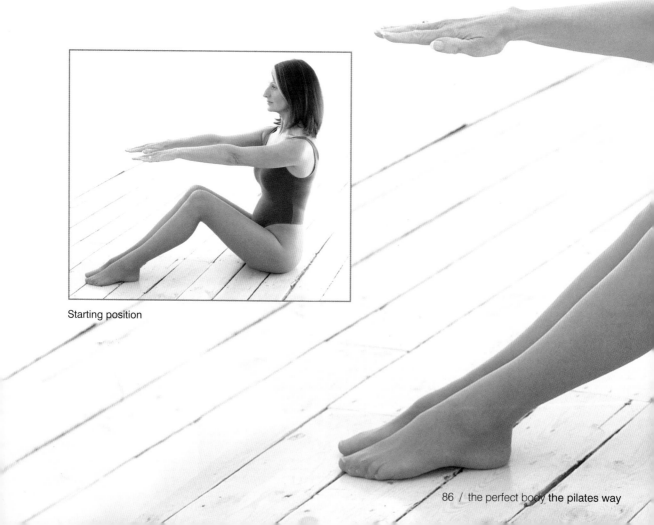

Starting position

6 Repeat five times to each side. You can help the rotation through the body by imagining that your straight arm is being pulled by a piece of string.

7 Repeat After this exercise come back into the Rest Position on page 54.

Watchpoints

- Keep zipping.
- Try not to tense your buttocks.
- Keep your neck released and feel the gap between the ears and the shoulders.

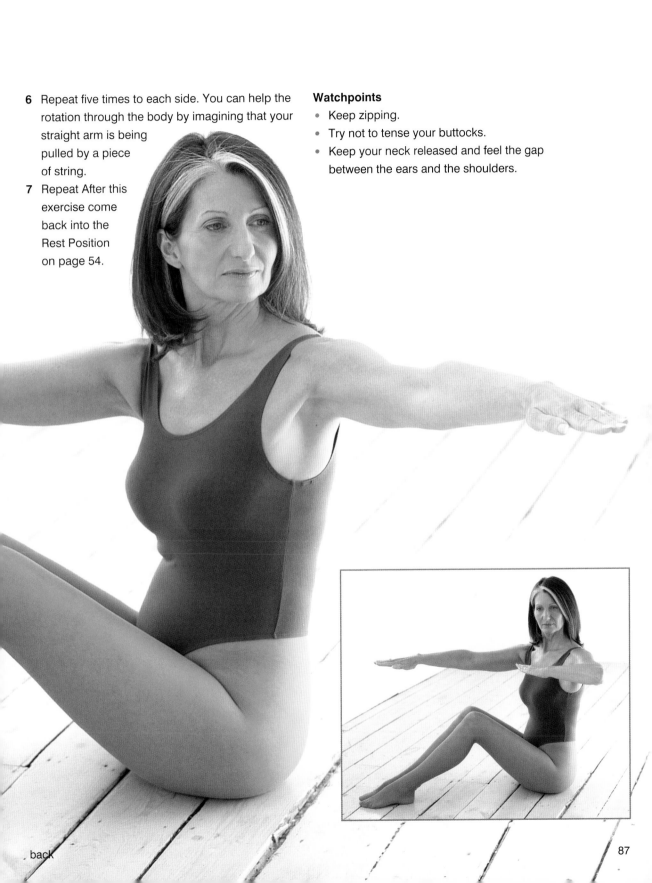

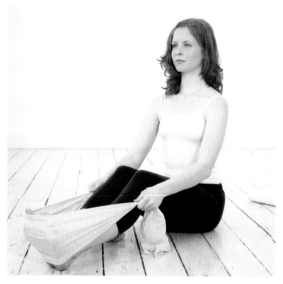

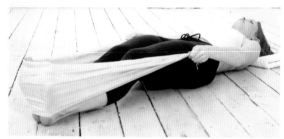

Starting position

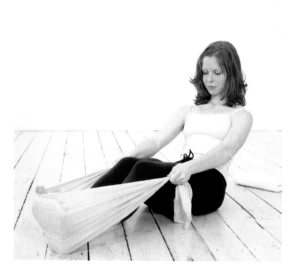

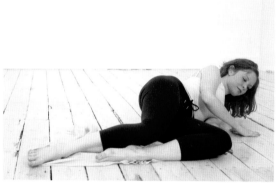

Getting in and out of position

Curl Downs (*advanced*)

A powerful exercise that tests both your core strength and the mobility of the spine.

The hip flexor muscles work in conjunction with the abdominal muscles, offering support to the front of the body. The fact that they are also attached to the spine gives them a role to play in the articulation of each vertebra – the wheeling movement we are constantly aiming for. It is important with these exercises to use the muscles in the most efficient sequence, for it is this that aids the mobilization of the spine. It demands that you relax certain muscles while focusing on and isolating others. If you allow your abdomen to bulge, then you are no longer using the right muscles, so be sure to keep hollowing.

This is a difficult exercise that must be performed with control. If you feel yourself coming down too fast, or if you feel any strain in your back, stop and wait until you are stronger and more flexible. When you are ready you could try coming down a third of the way and then coming back up again!

Aim
To strengthen the deep abdominals, thus promoting endurance. To learn to curl the spine, creating flexibility and strength.

Equipment
A long scarf or a stretchband. If you have a stretchband, use one with high resistance. A large towel or a flat cushion.

Starting Position
Sit on the floor with your knees bent, feet flat on the floor and together. Wrap the scarf around the feet. Put a folded towel or a flat cushion where your head will come to rest.

Action
1 Holding the scarf, breathe in and tilt your head forward so that your chin comes towards your chest but does not touch it.
2 Breathe out and zip up and hollow. Stay zipped throughout, and tilt the pelvis backwards so that the pubic bone comes up to meet your chin. Your tailbone remains on the floor, creating a C curve with the lumbar spine. Hollow your lower abdominals. Holding onto the scarf, slowly curl the back down to the floor, one vertebra at a time.
3 Remember to keep curling and hollowing. If your abdominals pop up, stop and try again when you are stronger.
4 Repeat up to ten times.
5 Each time you have finished curling down, sit up again in a normal, comfortable way – you may use your elbows or roll onto your side. Coming up isn't part of the exercise.

Watchpoints
- Stay in control.
- Keep your upper body relaxed and open, shoulder blades down into your back, neck released.

Back-rub Bliss

The power of touch can be truly overwhelming –
it strengthens the emotional bonds of friends and
family, invokes sensuality between partners and
boosts a sense of wellbeing in the individual.
When combined with simple massage techniques,
touch is particularly beneficial to the back, releasing
muscle tension and stimulating the circulation of
blood around the body.

Noella Gabriel, Treatment Development Director
for the esteemed aromatherapy company Elemis,
suggests these five easy ways to give a blissful
back massage. Choose one or combine several
techniques . . . just don't rush! Increase the benefits
by incorporating an aromatherapy massage oil –
you'll also find it makes the hands glide over the
back more fluidly. Pour a little into a small dish
and always start by dripping the oil up either side
of the spine.

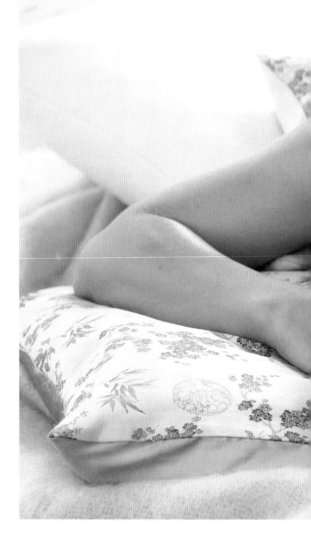

- Keeping the palms flat, start at the base of
  the back. Move the hands up along each side
  of the spine using a gentle pressure. As you
  reach the nape of the neck, move the hands
  across the wide part of the shoulders, then down
  the sides into the curves of the waist. Finish at the
  base of the back and repeat three or four times.
- Use the flat part of the thumbs – one following
  the other – to work up the right side of the spine
  from the base of the back to the nape of the neck.
  Applying firm pressure will help ease tight,
  knotted muscles. Continue out over the right
  shoulder, then repeat on the left side, starting
  from the base of the back.

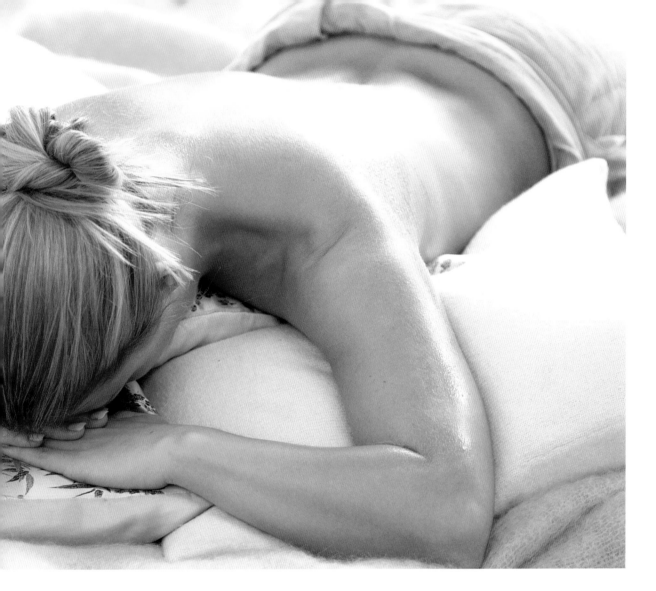

- Moving slowly all over the back, use both hands to gently pinch and roll the skin between the fingers and thumbs. This is ideal for stimulating and invigorating the body.
- Position yourself at the top of the head so you are looking down the body. Work along each side of the spine, from the nape of the neck to the base of the back in a circular movement, using the flat of the palms. Once you reach the lower back, use a kneading movement to help release tension.

- Again, positioning yourself at the top of the head, use the first three fingers of one hand to make deep circles around the right shoulder blade. Place the other hand on top of the first to increase the pressure and work out muscle knots (this area is usually very tight with tension). Repeat on the left side.

Skin Essentials

The skin on the back is prone to acne during puberty and often beyond. It can suffer from blocked pores if the skin is not cleansed thoroughly (especially after exercise) and, combined with a build-up of dead skin cells, this can mean spots and breakouts. Exfoliating at least once a week – be it with a loofah, a brush or a salt scrub – will give the skin a smooth, even texture. After just a few sessions of regular buffing, the back will be softer and more radiant.

Your exfoliator can be coarser than one you would use on the face as the skin is not as delicate on the body. Each of the methods below has its own merits – simply choose which will work best for you. Apply small circular movements but be gentle; you want to slough away dead skin, but not at the expense of being left red raw.

If you do suffer from spots or blemishes on your back, don't be over-zealous. Over-stimulating the skin can cause oil production and flare-ups to increase rather than diminish. Treat the skin gently and apply a mask or a mudpack once a week to draw out deep impurities and soak up excess oil.

Choose from these super smoothies:

Brushes, Loofahs, Cloths

A great way to slough off flaky patches, body brushes are made of natural bristles and best used on dry skin. This can feel slightly scratchy, but persevere because this technique is a great circulation booster too. One with a long, attachable handle is great for reaching the back. (For more details on this technique, turn to DIY Body Brushing on page 146.)

Loofahs are vegetables. They have a fibrous flesh that is dried out, but softens again when wet and can be used like a sponge all over the body to cleanse and buff. Exfoliating cloths are hugely popular in the East and are particularly practical for travelling as they take up little space and leave behind no residue. Simply smooth over the body in the bath or shower, concentrating on problem areas.

Salt Scrubs

These big chunky jars look great in the bathroom. The scrubs inside are usually a blend of sea salts and natural oils, pepped up with stimulating and reviving ingredients such as peppermint and ginger. They also have the benefit of dissolving in warm water which means that the granules won't stick to the skin but leave behind a soft sheen and a supple texture instead. Avoid them if you have oily skin.

Exfoliators

Body exfoliators are almost identical to those for your face, except the grains they contain are bigger and rougher, while the formulas are often richer and contain higher levels of foaming cleanser. A real no-brainer to use, simply apply the cream or gel all over the body and massage in. For an even easier option, switch from a manual scrub to a chemical version. These incorporate AHA fruit acids to smooth away even more dead cells while you shower, but may not be suitable for very sensitive skin.

Masks

To complete the back-care routine, team your buffing with a weekly body mask. These are rich and deep cleansing, drawing out the sebum, sweat, dead skin cells and dirt that clog pores and contribute to spots and blackheads. Some are made specifically for the body and have the added advantage of helping to feed it with skin-boosting minerals. However, if you want your face mask to double up for the back too, choose one that is clay or mud based and formulated for oily skins.

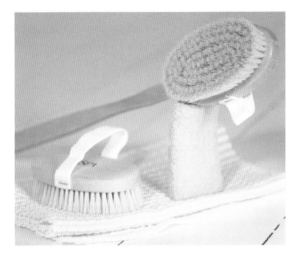

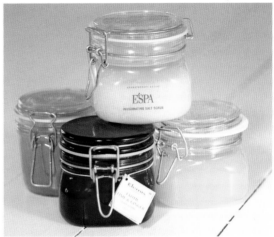

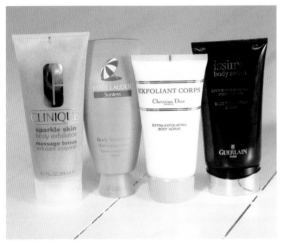

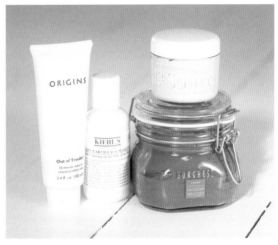

Brushes, Loofahs, Cloths

1 Elemis Skin Brush

2 Crabtree & Evelyn loofah

3 Space NK Japanese
  Body Cloth

4 E'SPA Skin Brush

Exfoliators

1 Clinique Sparkle Skin
  Body Exfoliator;

2 Estée Lauder Body Smoother
  Exfoliating Crème with AHAs

3 Christian Dior Extra
  Exfoliating Body Scrub

4 Guerlain Issima Body
  Secret Blue Exfoliating Scrub

Salt Scrubs

1 Elizabeth Arden Green Tea
  Tub Rub

2 E'SPA Invigorating Salt Scrub

3 Origins Salt Rub

4 Elemis Exotic Lime & Ginger
  Salt Glow

Masks

1 Origins Out of Trouble
  10-minute mask

2 Kiehl's Since 1851 Rare-Earth
  Face Masque

3 Crabtree and Evelyn La
  Source Deep Cleansing
  China Clay Mask

4 Borghese Fango Active Mud
  for Face and Body

THERE'S NO denying it – the simple truth is that if you take in more calories than you use, you will put on weight. But the way to a flatter, firmer tummy is not through crash diets but through eating a sensible balanced selection of food, consuming fewer calories than you burn while you are trying to lose weight and then eating just the right amount to stabilize your weight afterwards, combined with an effective exercise programme targeting and defining the abdominals and building lean muscle. In the meantime, there are some silhouette-slimming tricks you can learn too.

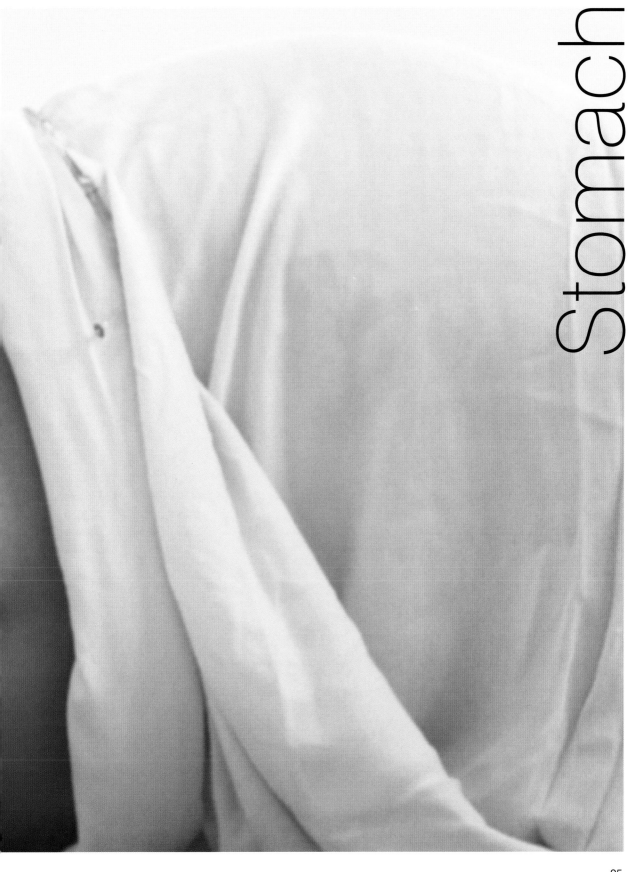

Stomach

Exercises for the Stomach Curl Ups (*beginners*)

You have four layers of abdominal muscles: rectus abdominis, commonly called the six-pack, is the most superficial; underneath these lie the external and internal obliques which criss-cross your torso defining your waistline; deepest of all, wrapping itself around you like a natural corset is the abdominal muscle Pilates' instructors love so much – the transversus abdominis. The problem with most types of stomach crunches and sit-ups is that in the search for the washboard effect they ignore the transversus. As a result the abdominals end up bulging as the exercise is performed and other muscles substitute and the flat stomach remains as elusive as ever. You must build your flat stomach on a solid foundation, strengthening from the inside out – from the core. Joseph Pilates called this area between the ribcage and the hips the powerhouse. Virtually all Pilates exercises use this powerhouse which means that in the course of one Pilates session you are doing hundreds of stomach exercises.

A few properly performed curl ups are worth hundreds of carelessly done sit-ups as the long, lean torsos of Pilates devotees will substantiate.

Aim
To strengthen the abdominals, engaging them in the correct order and with the trunk in perfect alignment. To achieve the ultimate flat stomach.

Starting Position
Lie in the Relaxation Position (see page 14). Clasp your hands behind your head; the elbows stay open.

Action
1   Breathe in, wide and full, to prepare.
2   Breathe out and zip up and hollow. Stay zipped throughout. Soften your breastbone, tuck your chin in a little and curl up, breaking from the breastbone.
3   Your stomach must not pop up. Keep the length and width in the front of the pelvis and the tailbone down on the floor lengthening away. Do not tuck the pelvis or pull on the neck.
4   Breathe in and slowly curl back down.
5   The aim is to get the shoulder blades clear of the mat, but only if the pelvis stays level.
6   Repeat ten times.

> **Warning:** avoid this exercise if you have neck problems.

Watchpoints

- Try not to grip around the hips.
- Stay in neutral, tailbone down on the floor and lengthening away. The front of the body keeps its length. A useful image is that there is a strip of sticky tape along the front of your body which should not wrinkle.
- Think of the ribcage funnelling down towards the waist.

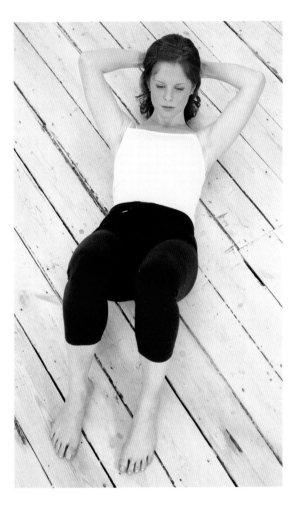

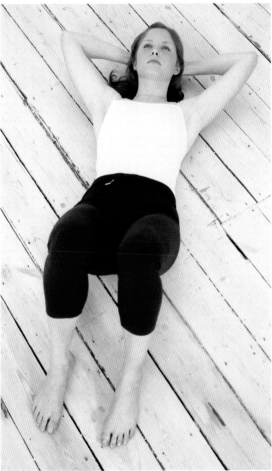

Starting position

Oblique Curl Ups (*beginners*)

It is the oblique muscles that give definition to the waist so if you are chasing an hourglass figure look for exercises that strengthen these muscles.

Aim

To work the obliques.

Starting Position

As for the previous exercise.

Action

1 Breathe in wide and full to prepare.
2 Breathe out and zip up and hollow. Stay zipped throughout, and bring your left shoulder across towards your right knee. The right elbow stays back. Your stomach must stay hollow, the pelvis stable.
3 Breathe in and lower.
4 Repeat five times to each side.

Watchpoints

- As for Curl Ups, make sure that the pelvis stays square and stable.
- Keep the upper body open.
- Keep the neck released.

> **Warning:** avoid this exercise if you have neck problems.

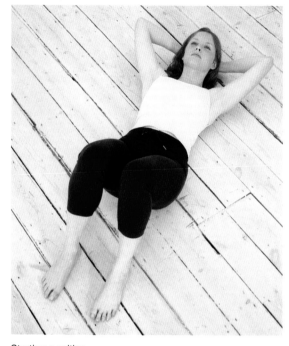

Starting position

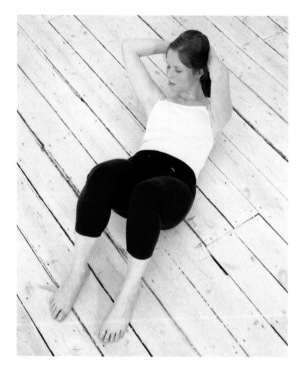

Hip Rolls (*beginners*)

Aim

To achieve rotation of the spine with stability.
To work the obliques (the waist).

Equipment

A tennis ball.

Starting Position

Lie in the Relaxation Position (see page 14).
Place your arms, palms up, out to the sides. Allow
the floor to support you. Allow your body to widen
and lengthen. Bring the feet together and place
a tennis ball between the knees. The tennis ball
ensures that the pelvis stays in good alignment.
It means that you have to work the waist that bit
harder to stay in line.

Action

1 Breathe in wide and full to prepare.
2 Breathe out and zip up and hollow. Roll your
   head in one direction, your knees in the other.
   Only roll a little way to start with – you can go
   further each time if it is comfortable. Keep your
   opposite shoulder down on the floor.

3 Breathe in, still zipping.
4 Breathe out and use your strong centre to
   bring the knees back to the starting position.
   The head comes back to the middle as well
5 Repeat eight times in each direction. Think of
   rolling each part of your back off the floor in
   sequence and then returning the back of the
   ribcage, the waist, the small of your back and
   the buttock to the floor.

Watchpoints

- Take care that you do not allow the back to arch.
- Keep working those abdominals. Do not simply
  allow the weight of the legs to pull you.
- The feet stay glued together alongside their
  inside edges but one foot will naturally come
  away from the floor as you roll to the side.

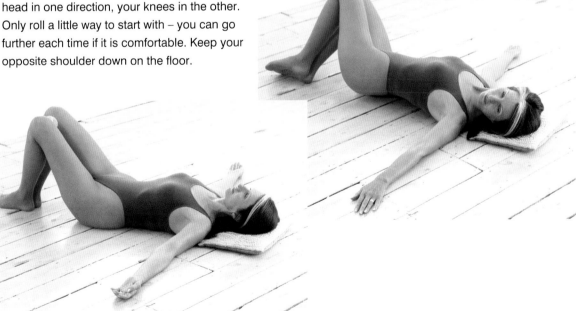

Starting position

Hip Rolls (*intermediate*)

Aim

To stretch and work the waist, strengthening the obliques. To achieve a safe rotation of the spine. To promote awareness of the shoulder blades, using the stabilizing muscles. To learn co-ordination skills.

We are looking here for rotation with stability. The ability to rotate the spine is the first movement we tend to lose as we grow older. There is a lot to think about with this exercise, which is great as we are trying to train the mind as well as the body. Focus on:

- Using the lower abdominals throughout.
- Peeling each part of your back off the floor in turn – first your buttocks leave the floor, then the hips, the waist and the back of the ribs. Then as you return to the centre, place each part back on the floor in reverse order – the ribs, the waist, the hips, the buttocks.
- As you turn the palm down, think of the shoulder blade setting itself down into your back.

Equipment

A tennis ball.

Starting Position

Lie on your back, arms out to the side, palms up. Zip up and hollow and bring the knees up one at a time so that they are above your hips. Place the tennis ball between your knees. Your thighs will be at right angles to your body. Your feet are softly pointed.

Action

1 Breathe in wide and full to prepare. As you breathe out, zip up and hollow, and slowly lower your legs towards the floor on your right side, turning your head to the left and your left palm down. Keep the left shoulder down on the ground. Keep the knees in line.
2 Breathe in and breathe out, still zipped and hollowed, and use this strong centre to bring your legs back to the middle. The head also returns to the middle, the palm turns up again.
3 Breathe in and then out, and repeat the twisting movement to the opposite side.
4 Repeat ten times to each side.

Watchpoints

- Keep the opposite shoulder firmly down on the floor.
- Keep the knees in line. Don't go too far unless you can control them.
- Use the abdominals at all times – feel as though you are moving the legs from the stomach.
- This is a sideways lateral movement – don't deviate.
- Do not force the neck the opposite way, allow it to roll comfortably and keep it long.

> **Warning:** please take advice if you have a disc-related injury.

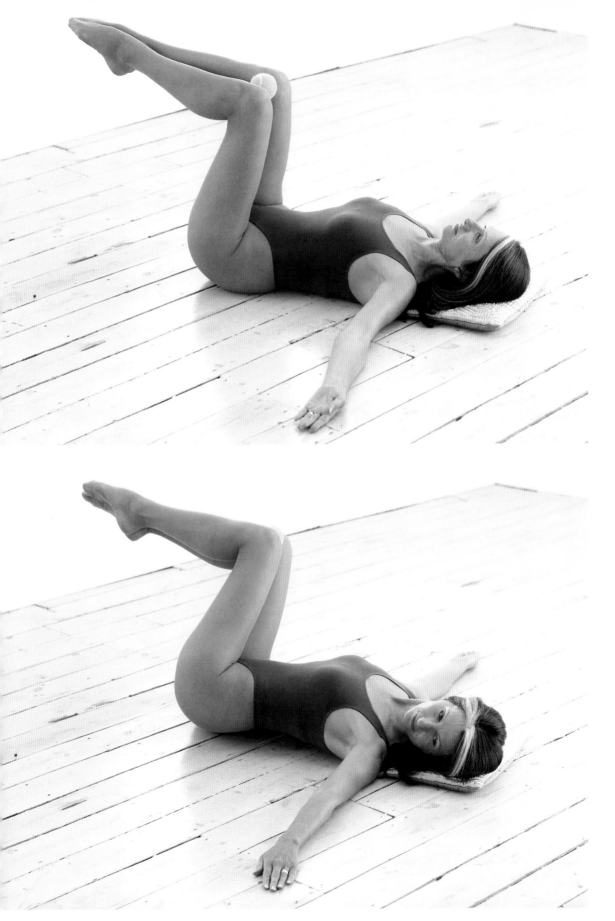

Single Leg Stretch *Level One* (*beginners*)

Aim

This is a classical Pilates exercise which is best taught in simple stages. It challenges both the abdominals and your co-ordination. In fact, it combines *all* the Eight Principles.

Starting Position

Lie in the Relaxation Position (see page 14).

Action

1 Breathe in wide and full to prepare.
2 Breathe out, zip up and hollow, and fold one knee at a time up to your chest.
3 Breathe in and grasp your right knee with both hands. Keep your elbows open and your breastbone soft. Your shoulder blades stay down into your back. Neck released.
4 Breathe out, zip up and hollow, and slowly straighten the left leg straight up into the air. Keep your back anchored into the floor.

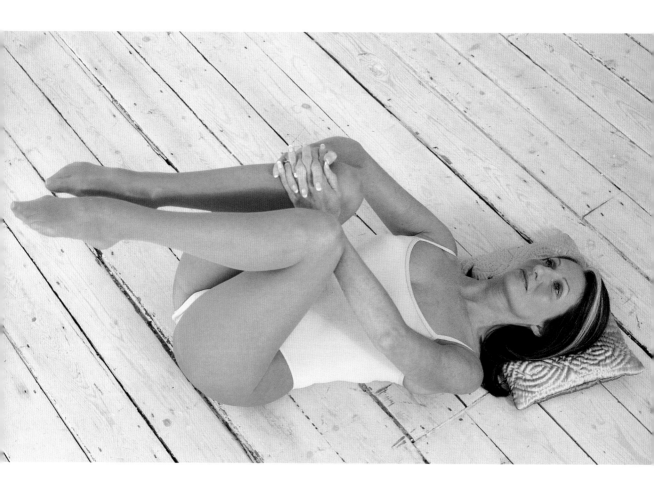

5 Breathe in and bend the knee back in. Change hands and repeat with the other leg.

6 Repeat ten times with each leg. Do not allow the leg to fall away from you. Your back must stay anchored to the floor. When this becomes easy – and only then – you may try the more advanced version on page 104.

Watchpoints

- Keep your actions smooth and flowing.
- Stay in neutral.
- The lower the extended leg goes, the harder your abdominals work – keep the leg high.

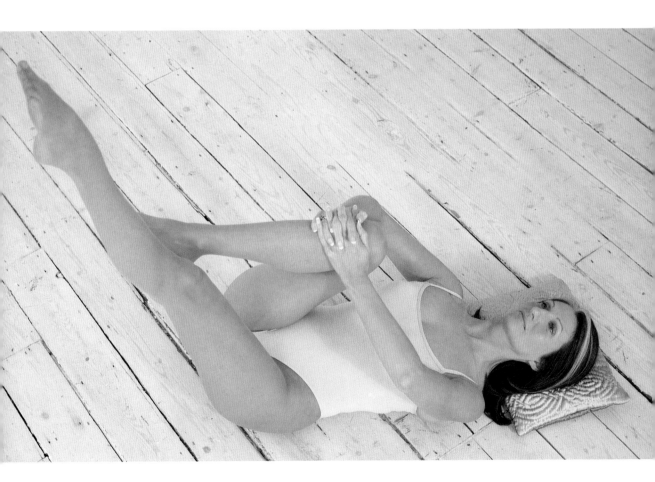

Single Leg Stretch *Level Two* (*intermediate*)

This has to be the best abdominal exercise there is. You might like to practise the arm movements separately before attempting the full version – they are quite challenging.

Arm Movement

- Sit tall on the floor with your knees bent in front of you.
- Place the right hand on the outside of the right calf, the left hand on the inside of the right knee.
- Change hands: left hand on the outside of the left calf, right hand on the inside of the left knee. So – outside calf; inside knee.
- This keeps the upper body open and relaxed and enables you to breathe fully.

Starting Position

Lie in the Relaxation Position (see page 14).

Action

1 Breathe in to prepare.
2 Breathe out, zip up and hollow, and fold your knees up to your chest one at a time. Keep your feet softly pointed. Place your hands on the outside of your calves.
3 Breathe in. Check that your elbows are open to enable the chest to expand fully. Your shoulder blades are down into your back.
4 Breathe out, zip up and hollow, soften your breastbone and curl the upper body off the floor.
5 Breathe in and place the right hand on the outside of the right calf, the left hand on the inside of the right knee.
6 Breathe out and, zipping up and hollowing, slowly stretch your left leg away, so that it is at an angle of about 45° to the floor. The toes are softly pointed.
7 Breathe in wide and full, as you begin to bend the leg back to your chest.
8 Change the hands so that your left hand is on the outside of your left calf, your right hand on the inside of your left knee.
9 Breathe out and, still zipping and hollowing, stretch the right leg away. Do not take it too close to the floor.
10 Breathe in as the leg returns.
11 Repeat ten stretches with each leg, making sure that you have a strong centre throughout and that your shoulder blades stay down into your back, and your elbows are open.

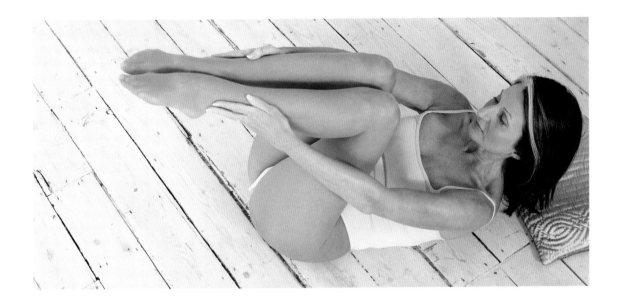

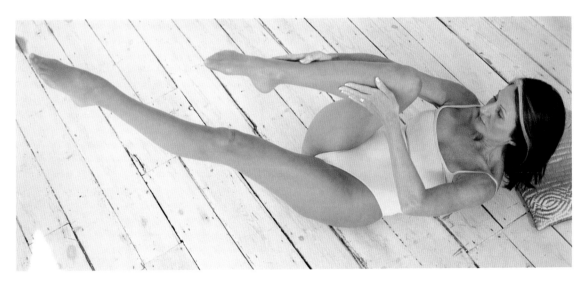

Watchpoints

- Keep zipping and hollowing throughout and do not allow the back to arch. The pelvis stays neutral.
- Keep your neck released and your upper body open, shoulder blades down.

- Make sure that you keep the length on both sides of your waist, do not allow one side to shorten.
- Raise the extended leg higher if you feel that your back is arching.

Criss-Cross (*advanced*)

A powerful exercise that hits the spot. You'll need strong abdominals to do this one correctly.

Aim

To work the abdominals – especially the obliques – while challenging co-ordination and core stability.

Starting Position

Lie on your back in the Relaxation Position (see page 14). Zip up and hollow, and draw your knees up to your chest one at a time; have the toes just touching, but not the heels. Keep your feet softly pointed. Clasp your hands behind your head. The elbows stay open.

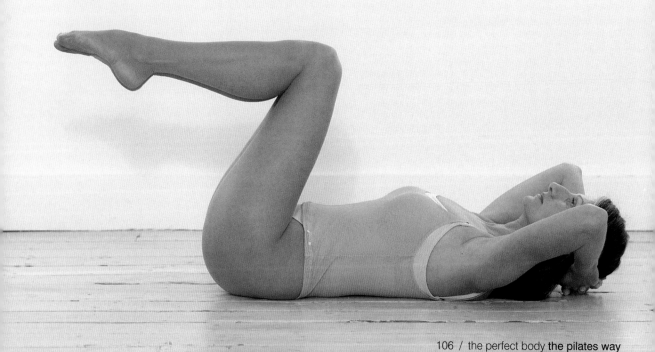

Action

1 Breathe in wide and full to prepare.

2 Breathe out and zip up and hollow as you curl up, softening the breastbone and taking the right shoulder in the direction of your left knee. The upper body stays open, the elbows in line. At the same time straighten the right leg, extending it in parallel at an angle of about 45° to the floor.

3 Breathe out, still zipped and hollowed, bend the right leg back toward the chest and curl the left shoulder towards the bent right knee while extending the left leg away.

4 Repeat ten times to each side.

Watchpoints

- Do not bring the elbows together towards your ears – keep them open.
- Stay neutral please.

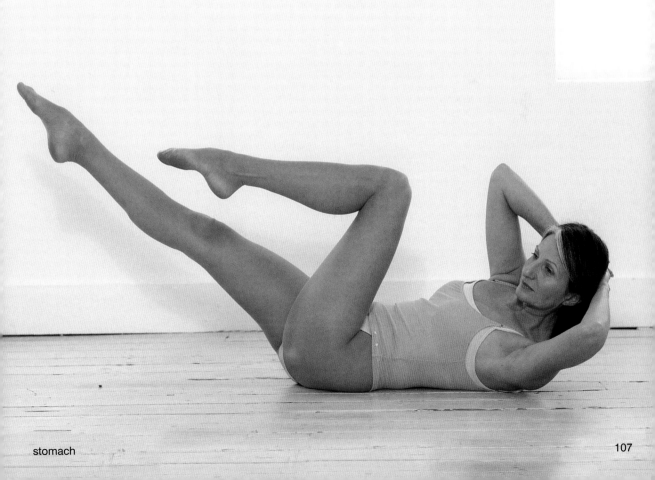

See-Saw *Level One (intermediate)*

There are two levels to this wonderful exercise which is great for strengthening your powerhouse.

Aim

To work the muscles of the trunk while dynamically stretching the legs.

Starting Position

Sit tall on your sitting bones with your knees bent in front of you, feet flat on the floor. Clasp your hands behind your thighs. Now you have a choice. This exercise can be done maintaining the natural curve of the spine or by adopting a C-curve with the lower back. For a C-shaped spine gently roll back the pelvis, supporting your spine with your lower abdominals. Think of opening the low back but do not collapse; keep lengthening upwards. You must decide which feels more comfortable for you. Either way, your shoulder blades stay down into your back, your elbows open and your neck released.

Action

1 Breathe in wide and full and lengthen through the spine.
2 Breathe out and zip up and hollow. Stay zipped throughout, and slowly straighten one leg. Lengthen through the leg.
3 Breathe in and bend the knee.
4 Repeat three times with each leg.

Watchpoints

- Only straighten the leg as far as you are comfortable. This exercise requires length in the hamstrings.
- Stay zipped!
- Keep lengthening up through the spine.

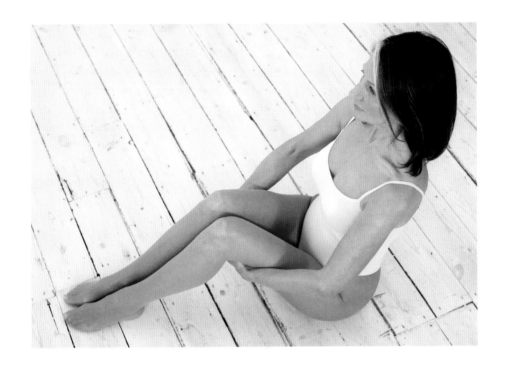

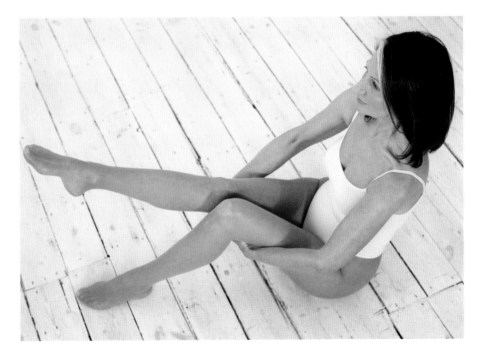

stomach

See-Saw *Level Two (advanced)*

A more challenging version.

Starting Position

Lie back on your elbows, fingertips facing forwards, palms down. Your knees are bent up to your chest. You will be balancing on your sitting bones at the bottom of your pelvis. Do not sink down; lengthen through the spine, shoulder blades down into your back. Keep the distance between your ears and your shoulders.

Action

1 Breathe in wide and full to prepare.
2 Breathe out and zip up and hollow. Stay zipped throughout, and slowly and with control straighten both legs away from you. Use the momentum of this action to come up on to your hands, with the elbows straightening at the same time as the legs. The finished position is to be balancing on the sitting bones, legs extended at an angle of about 45°, elbows straight but not locked. A see-saw action.

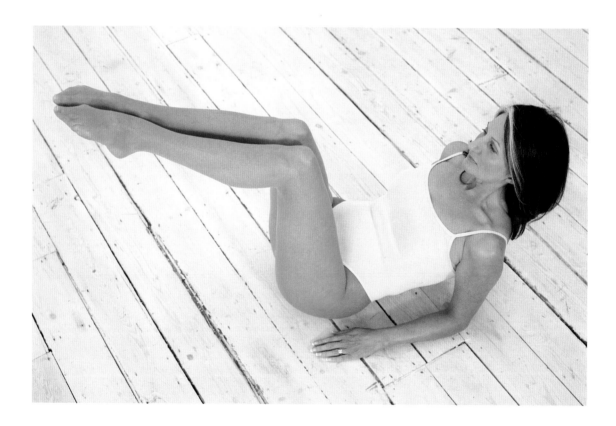

3 Breathe in and come back on to the elbows, bending the knees again.

4 Repeat five times.

Watchpoints

- Control the movement: keep it smooth and flowing.
- Try to push up evenly on both arms.
- When the legs are extended, lengthen through the toes: long, long legs, strong centre. At the same time, lengthen through the top of the head.

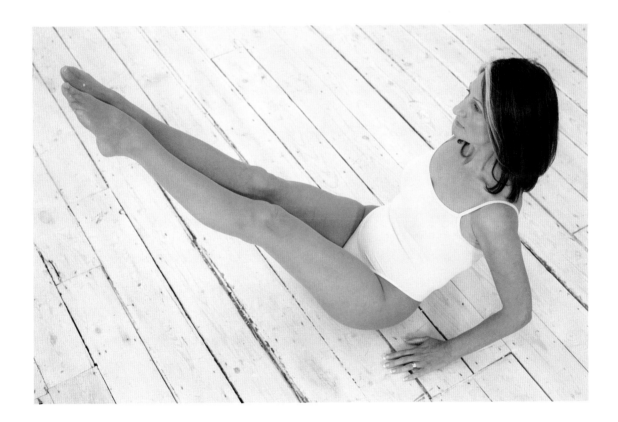

Scissors (*beginners*)

A great exercise for the stomach and the legs.

Aim

To work the abdominals. To learn how to hinge the leg from the hip joint.

Starting Position

Lie in the Relaxation Position (see page 14). Zip up and hollow, and bring your knees up to your chest one at a time. Take hold of the left knee with both hands and hold it securely to you. Keep the elbows open, the neck soft and the shoulder blades down into your back. Stay in the neutral pelvis position throughout the exercise.

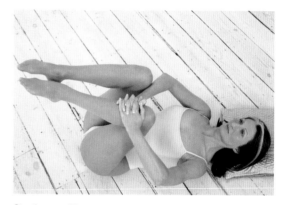

Starting position

Action

1 Breathe in wide and full.
2 Breathe out and zip up and hollow. Stay zipped throughout, and straighten the right leg up into the air.
3 Breathe in and flex the right foot down towards your face, lengthening through the heel.
4 Keep the leg straight, foot flexed.
5 Breathe out and lower the straight leg to the floor, lengthening the whole time through the heel . . . a long, long leg.
6 Breathe in as the foot rests on the floor and then out again as you raise the leg.
7 Repeat eight times on each leg.

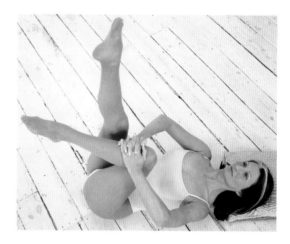

Watchpoints

• Try to hinge the leg from the hip joint.
• Stay in neutral pelvis.
• Keep your elbows open, your breastbone soft and your neck released.

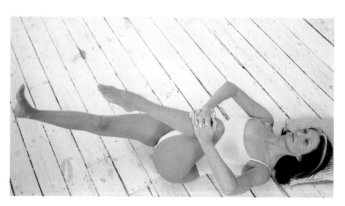

Scissors (*intermediate*)

Aim

To strengthen the abdominals, improve co-ordination and promote the flexibility of the hamstrings.

Starting Position

Lie in the Relaxation Position (see page 20). Zip up and hollow, and bring your knees up to your chest. Take hold of the right leg behind the thigh.

Action

1 Breathe in wide and full to prepare.
2 Breathe out and zip up and hollow. Stay zipped throughout, and curl the head and shoulders off the mat. Keep the breastbone soft.
3 Breathe in and straighten both legs up into the air, toes softly pointed. You are still holding the right leg behind the thigh.
4 Breathe out and lengthen the left leg towards the floor, stopping just above it.
5 Breathe in and raise the leg as straight as possible.
6 Breathe out and change arms and legs, lowering the right leg now.
7 Repeat ten times on each leg, aiming to cross over like scissors.

Watchpoints

- Keep zipping and hollowing throughout, pelvis neutral, the tailbone lengthening away. The full version requires very strong abdominals.
- The upper body stays soft and open, your shoulder blades are down into your back.
- Keep your legs as straight as possible – long, long legs.
- Keep your actions smooth, flowing and controlled.

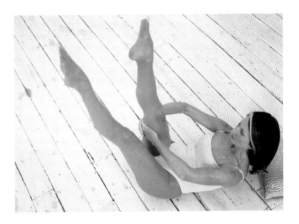

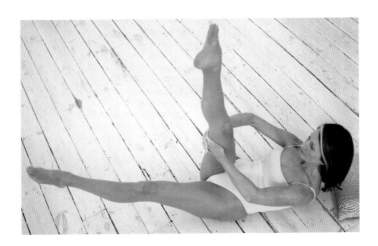

stomach

Torpedo (*intermediate*)

Aim

To work the obliques and to test your core stability, balance and alignment. This is a real waist-whittler.

Starting Position

Lie in a straight line on your side – shoulder over shoulder, hip over hip, your legs stretched out in a line with your body. Extend your lower arm along the floor above your head, which rests on it, in line with your torso; the top arm bends in front of you to support you. Your hand will be in a line with your chest, your shoulder blade down into the back, elbow open.

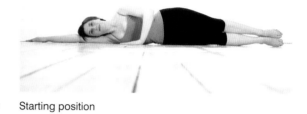

Starting position

Action

1 Breathe out and zip up and hollow.
2 Breathe in and keep zipping as you lift both legs together off the mat.
3 Breathe out and raise the upper leg higher, staying parallel with the lower leg. Feel the length of the body from fingertip to toes, long and strong.
4 Breathe in, lower the top leg to the lower leg.
5 Breathe out and gently lower both legs back to the floor.
6 Repeat five times to each side.

Watchpoints

• Try not to use the supporting arm to push yourself up.
• Make sure you maintain neutral pelvis and spine. Do not arch the back.
• Keep an open elbow on the supporting arm, the shoulder stays down.
• Really enjoy the lengthening through the whole body, keeping a long waistline.

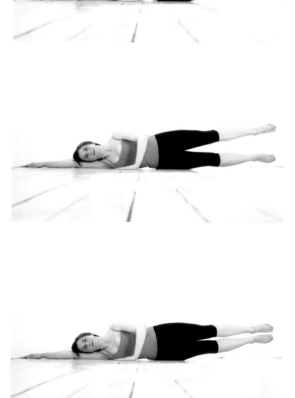

Front Leg Pull (*advanced*)

A challenging exercise that requires good upper-body strength as well as good core strength.

Aim
This exercise really challenges the powerhouse, and conditions the whole body.

Starting Position
Adopt a traditional push-up position, making sure that your body is long and the shoulders are drawn down into your back. The fingers point forward, the elbows stay straight but not locked, head in line with the body, legs hip-width apart. You should feel as if your body is being pulled in two directions.

Action
1   Breathe in to prepare.
2   Breathe out and zip up and hollow. Stay zipped throughout, and press the heels away from you. Think of a plank of wood or an ironing board.
3   Breathe in as you lift one leg (keeping the foot flexed) towards the ceiling without moving the hips or allowing the back to arch. Keep lengthening the head away and keep the ribcage flat.
4   Breathe out as you lower the leg back to the floor still lengthening through the heel.
5   Repeat five times with each leg.

Watchpoints
* Keep your shoulder blades connected down into your back.
* Keep the back of the neck long and released.
* Don't dip in the middle.

> **Warning:** avoid this exercise if you have shoulder problems.

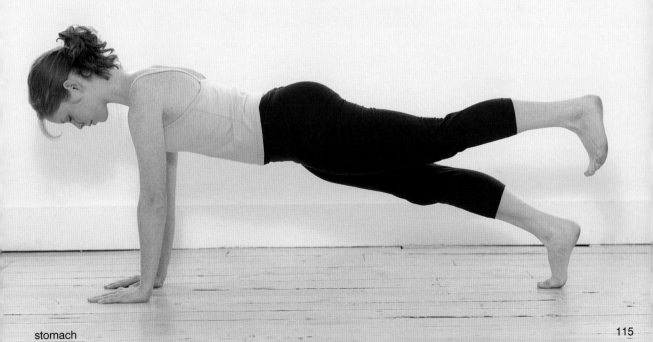

stomach

Eating for a Flatter Stomach

Many of us overeat or eat foods that fool the body into thinking it is still hungry – in both cases the stomach can distend while the extra calories consumed lead to excess weight. A varied and healthy eating plan (outlined in Eating to Fight Fat on page 138) is essential for a balanced body shape and a sleeker silhouette, but you also need to ensure that your digestive system is working at its optimum.

Inside the stomach are tiny receptors that send messages to the brain when they are stretched, letting it know that the stomach feels full. Certain foods – those low in fibre – are less bulky and so don't cause the receptors to stretch quite as quickly as bulkier, fibre-rich foods. The result is that you will want to eat more, or more often. In addition, eating the wrong foods too quickly can bloat the stomach (as can PMT for women), which can be uncomfortable and make you feel unattractive. There is also the more controversial issue of food intolerance – some nutritionists believe that many of us suffer from intolerance to common foods such as wheat and dairy products. If this is the case, such foods may also bloat the stomach. If you feel you have an intolerance to a particular food, experiment and see what happens after you eat it – you may see a pattern and be able to work out for yourself what is happening. If not, seek the advice of a qualified professional.

Any time you eat or drink the stomach is naturally going to expand, but combining a healthy meal plan with these clever eating tips will help keep bloating to a minimum.

- Eat slowly, taking small mouthfuls of your food and sips of your drink and chewing well. The brain takes fifteen minutes to receive the message that your stomach has had enough to eat, so eating too quickly will result in overeating. Meanwhile, gulping can cause excess air to fill the stomach, contributing to a bloated appearance.
- Give your food your full attention. Not concentrating on what you are eating means you are more likely to miss those signals saying you are full.
- At meal times, relax but keep good posture as you sit. Not only can the body then concentrate on digesting food (rather than moving about or pumping adrenalin, for example), but the internal organs are in the best position to do so.
- Change your eating patterns so that you have smaller meals more frequently. This way, the stomach doesn't have to cope with two or three large intakes of food every day.
- Keep your intake of salty foods to a minimum as these can encourage fluid retention, especially in women in the days leading up to the start of menstruation.
- Having fizzy drinks with meals will increase the chances of wind and heartburn.
- Try not to eat the same food two days running (notice how difficult this is). This way you can help ensure that you have a varied diet and could also help to prevent building food intolerances.
- Some people find fruit easier to digest if it is eaten at least an hour before or after a meal.

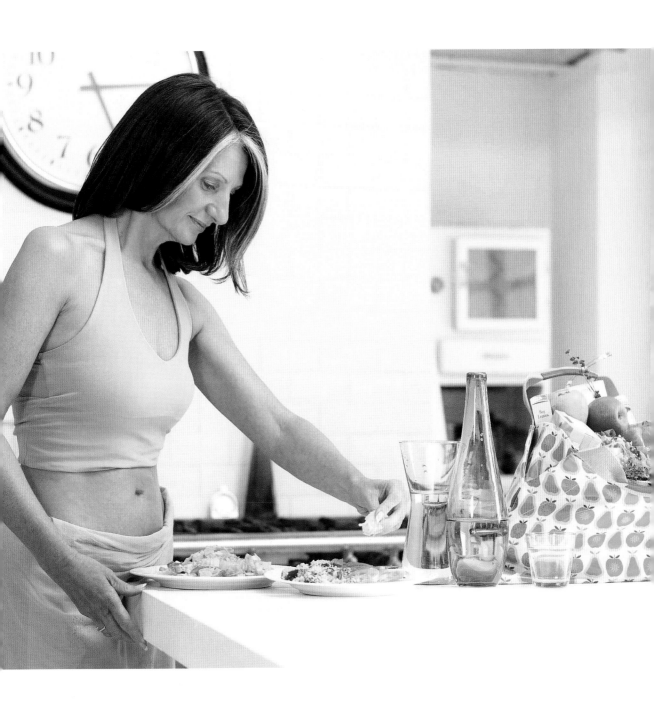

stomach

Foods to Stock Up On

- Fresh herbs and spices: coriander eases flatulence; cumin and cloves assist digestion; sorrel helps prevent stomach aches. Herbal infusions such as peppermint, camomile, lemon balm and fennel all calm and soothe the digestive system, helping to remedy bloating and wind. Sip a cup between meals.
- High-fibre foods: including pulses, fresh vegetables, wholegrain bread and pasta. These swell and take longer for the body to digest, so the receptors in the stomach ensure that it feels fuller for longer. You therefore need to eat less and less often.
- Broccoli, kidney beans and sunflower seeds: rich in vitamin B6 which is needed to produce the digestive enzymes that break down food in the intestines.
- Pre- and probiotics: prebiotics such as bananas, asparagus and artichokes, encourage the growth of beneficial bacteria in the digestive system, which fight infections such as thrush. Probiotics such as live yoghurt are themselves rich in these good bacteria.

Stay-svelte Tea

Not only is fennel a traditional remedy for indigestion, it is often used to help reduce water retention. Because of its diuretic properties, sweet fennel tea effectively flushes excess fluids and toxins from the body, especially in women who are pre-menstrual. After overindulging in a heavy meal, sipping a cup can also ease bloating and wind.

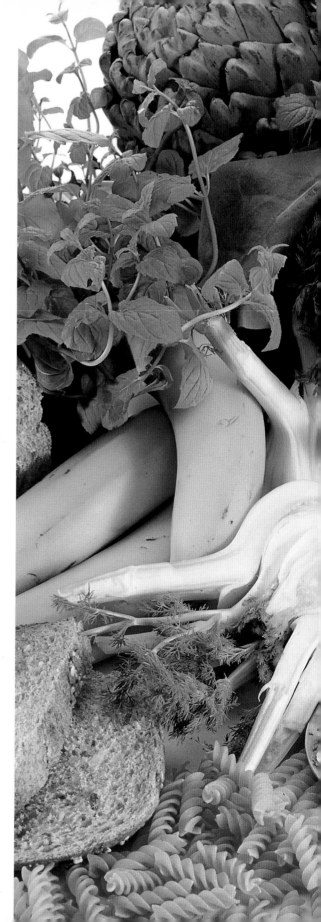

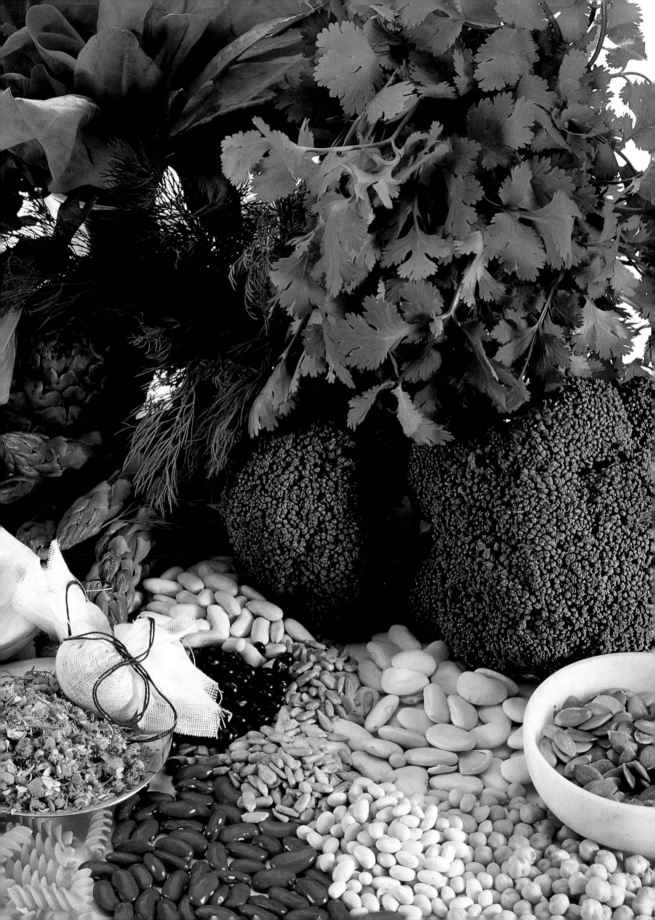

Penne with Artichokes and Lemon

Preparation time: **15 minutes**
Cooking time: **30 minutes**
Serves: **2**

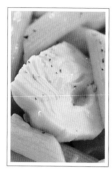

200g penne or other dried pasta
4 tbsp olive oil
1 clove garlic, crushed
400g can artichoke hearts in water,
    rinsed, drained and sliced in half
juice and zest of 1 lemon
salt and freshly ground black pepper

Cook the pasta according to the instructions.

Heat 1 tbsp of the olive oil in a non-stick pan, add the garlic and artichokes and cook for 3–4 minutes.

Whisk the lemon juice and zest with the remaining olive oil.

Drain the pasta and transfer to a warm serving bowl. Stir in the artichoke hearts, olive oil and lemon juice. Season to taste and serve.

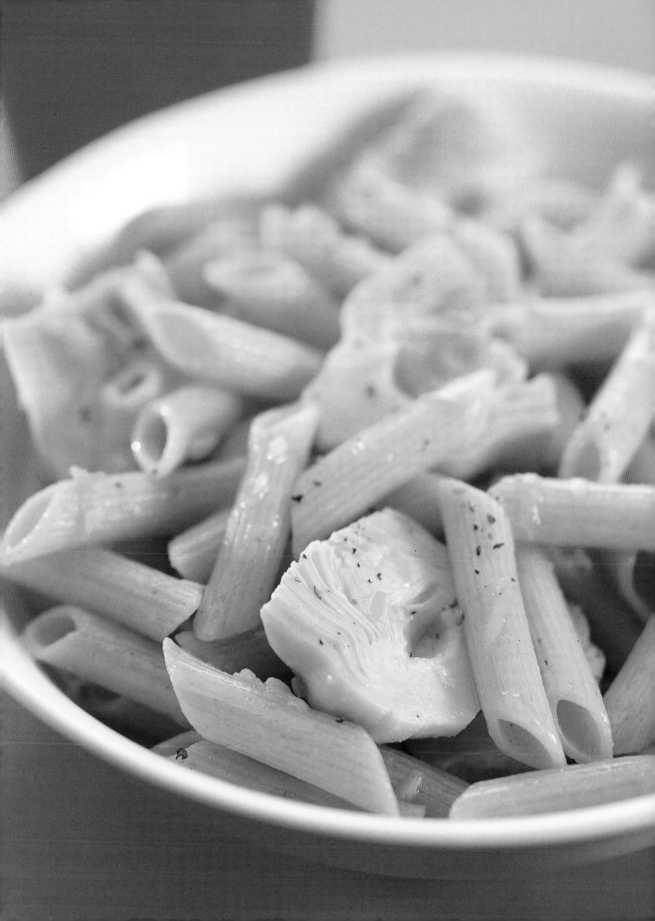

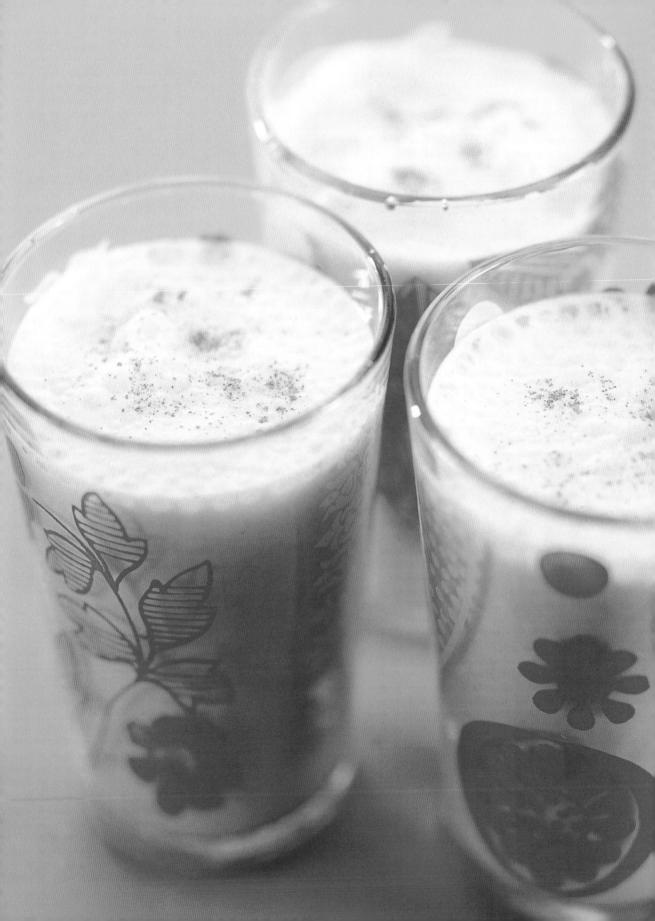

Banana and Almond Smoothie

Preparation time: **5 minutes, plus 2 hours freezing**
Cooking time: **nil**
Serves: **1**

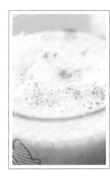

1 ripe banana, sliced

250ml skimmed milk

25g ground almonds

pinch of ground cinnamon

a little honey to sweeten (optional)

Put the banana into a freezer-proof container and freeze
for at least 2 hours or overnight.

Place all the ingredients in a blender or food processor
and blend until thick and frothy. Pour into a glass and
serve immediately.

Cheers! The Pros and Cons of Alcohol

While over-indulging on a regular basis is bad for the body both inside and out, a small tipple now and again can do more good than harm. The key is moderation.

The Pros

In the past few years, a vast amount of medical research has been done on the effects of alcohol on the body. Recent results have shown that a moderate amount of alcohol every day (say, one small glass of wine) can actually help reduce the risk of coronary heart disease. This is because many alcoholic drinks – red wine in particular – contain antioxidants that reduce the amount of artery-clogging cholesterol in the blood.

The mild relaxing effect also helps lower blood pressure and stress levels, and this plays a part in keeping the heart healthy. In addition, red wine may help prevent blood clots and Alzheimer's in older people. However, these benefits can only be felt if the recommended number of units per week is broken up into small amounts (2–3 units per day), rather than a one-night binge.

The Cons

Exceeding the recommended number of units per week can have serious health risks including liver damage, high blood pressure and heart problems. Long term, it can also diminish sexual desire and ability.

Excessive drinking isn't good for the appearance either. As well as weight gain (one gram of alcohol contains 7 calories; one unit contains 8 grams of alcohol), the dehydrating effects cause the skin to become dry and flaky, while nutritional deficiency means that the body cannot absorb some of the vitamins (B and C), minerals (zinc) and fats (essential fatty acids) necessary for a healthy, glowing complexion. Alcohol is a depressant, and after its initial stimulating effects it can make you drowsy, but then it tends to prevent rather than to encourage sleep, disrupting sleep patterns so that you look and feel tired the day following a binge.

Drinking on an empty stomach and drinks with 'fizz', such as champagne or spirits with carbonated mixers, encourage alcohol to enter the bloodstream more quickly, meaning you feel the effects faster. When you do drink, match each glass of alcohol with a glass of water to help stave off ill effects the following morning.

Raise a Glass

Mixers, such as carbonated drinks, contain a large amount of sugar, significantly increasing your calorie intake, so opt for the diet versions.

One alcoholic drink can conceal a surprising number of calories too.

small glass dry white wine (125ml) = 1 unit of alcohol = 83 calories

small glass red wine (125ml) = 1 unit = 85 calories

glass of champagne (125ml) = 1 unit = 95 calories

single measure of spirits (25 ml) = 1 unit = 52 calories

pint of beer or lager = 2 units = 167 calories

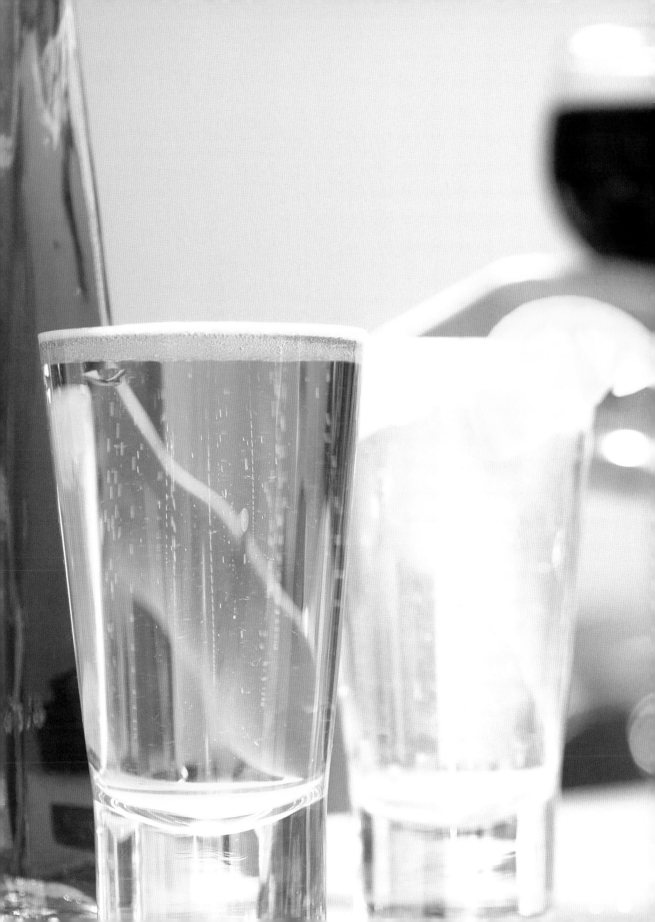

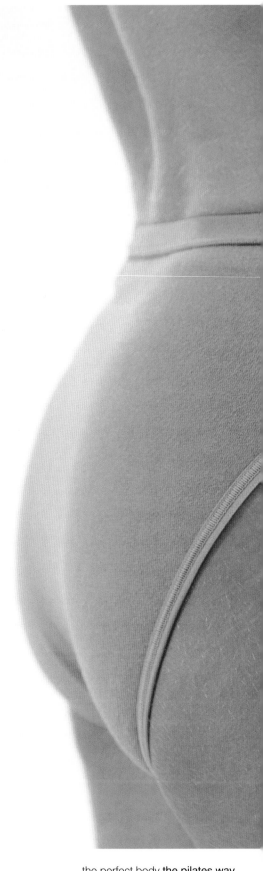

U NDER COVER
and out of sight, the
buttocks are the area
of the body that need most
but usually receive the least
attention. Couch-potato
culture means that we spend
most of the day sitting on
them, either at work or at
home – a lifestyle that only
encourages sluggish
circulation and fatty deposits.
A healthy diet plays a key
part in fighting fat, but adding
the right Pilates exercises
and an easy beauty routine
will ensure a tight, toned
bottom with peachy soft skin.

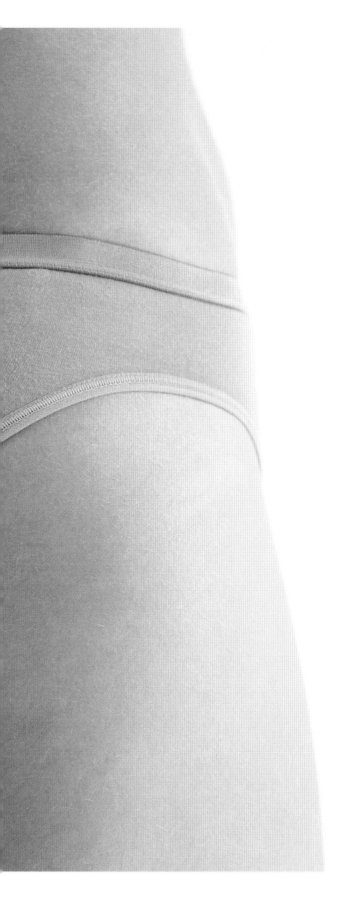

Bottom

Exercises for the Buttocks Oyster (*beginners*)

You have three buttock muscles: gluteus maximus, medius and minimus. The gluteus maximus muscle is the largest muscle in the body – and often the least toned. Sitting on it all day does not help. Make the decision to take the stairs rather than the lift or escalator, walk rather than take transport and you will quickly see a difference, but if you want to really firm up you will need exercises that isolate the gluteals.

If you want to feel where your deep gluteals lie then this is the exercise to show you. It targets the gluteus medius muscle which is crucial in stabilizing the pelvis. That's the medical reason why you should do it – the cosmetic reason is that it tightens your butt!

Aim
To strengthen the gluteus medius. It is also a very good exercise if you have knee problems as it helps to correct the muscle imbalances that sometimes cause these.

Equipment
A flat pillow (optional).

Starting Position
Lie in a straight line on your side. Have your underneath arm stretched out in a line with your body and place a flat pillow between your ear and arm so that your neck keeps a line with your spine. Bend your knees, keeping your feet in a line with your bottom.

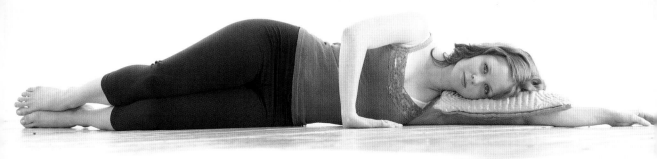

Action

1 Breathe in wide and full to prepare.

2 Breathe out and zip up and hollow. Stay zipped throughout, and slowly rotate your top leg, opening the knee. Make sure as you do so that you do not lose your neutral pelvis or spine, and keep lengthening through the body. Your feet stay on the floor together. The movement begins in the buttocks.

3 Breathe in and hold.

4 Breathe out and close.

5 Repeat up to ten times on each side.

Watchpoints

- Try to feel as though you are drawing the thigh bone back into the hip socket; the action is quite subtle but very powerful.
- Do not allow the waist to sink into the floor, keep it long.
- Do not allow your pelvis to roll backward or your upper body to fall forward.
- Maintain a neutral pelvis throughout.

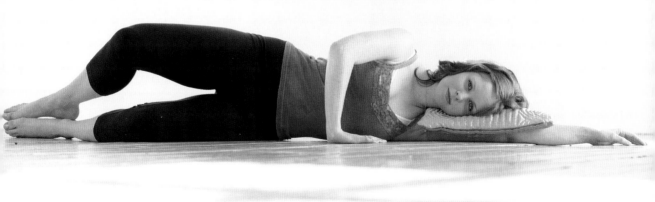

bottom

Buttock Walking (*beginners*)

Legend has it that Grace Kelly used to do this exercise to keep her bottom trim. And if you are too young to remember who Grace Kelly was, she was a Hollywood legend who married a prince – so clearly it worked for her! It isn't really a Pilates exercise, but it works brilliantly.

Aim

To strengthen the buttock muscles and keep cellulite at bay. Unfortunately, a hard surface works better than a soft one so the floor is a good option.

Starting Position

Sit tall on your sitting bones with your legs stretched out in front of you. Cross your arms so that you are holding your opposite shoulder lightly.

Action

1 Breathe in wide and full and lengthen through the spine.
2 Breathe out, zip up and hollow. Stay zipped throughout, breathing normally as you shuffle forwards across the floor and then back again.
3 Repeat as often as you can!

Watchpoints

- Try to avoid nylon carpet (carpet burn), coir matting (grazing) or old wooden floors (splinters).
- Keep tall as you shuffle.

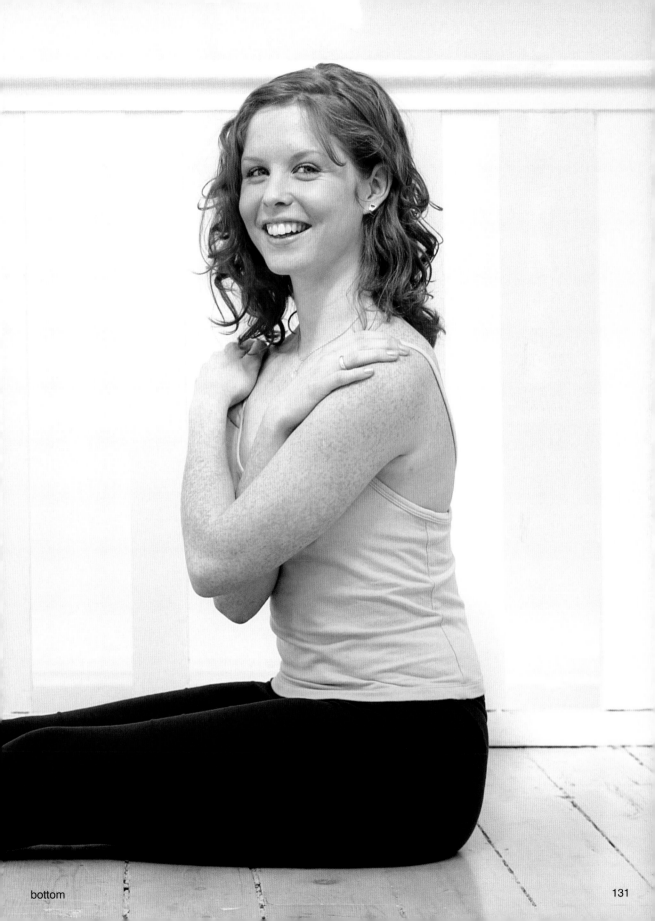

One-legged Knee Bends Barre Exercise (*beginners*)

Don't let the long name put you off, it really hits
the spot.

These traditional barre exercises are a great
workout for the legs and buttocks and are proof that
you do not need expensive elaborate equipment to
get real results fast.

Aim

To strengthen the leg muscles, thighs, calves and
buttocks. To learn correct alignment of the legs.
To achieve pelvic stability.

You must also pay close attention to your pelvis.
It must stay level as you bend the knee.

Starting Position

Stand with your right side to the wall, or a chair,
remembering to lengthen up through the spine.
Bend the right leg, so that the knee faces straight
forward and the foot is resting just beside the other
knee. Hold onto the wall or the chair.

Action

1 Breathe in and lengthen up through the spine.
2 Breathe out, zip up and hollow, and rise up onto
   your toes.
3 Breathe in.

4 Breathe out, still zipped and hollowed, and
   slowly bring your left heel back down to the floor.
   Think of the heel lengthening away from the top
   of your head. It is as if your head stays up there.
5 Now breathe in wide and full.
6 Breathe out, still zipped and hollowed, and bend
   your left knee, bringing the kneecap directly over
   the centre of your foot. As you do so, do not sink
   into your hips, keep lengthening up and keep
   your pelvis level.
7 Breathe in and straighten the leg; see if you can
   think of pulling up the thigh muscles as you do so.
8 Repeat five times on each leg, turning round
   so that your bent knee side is to the wall. Do not
   allow your bottom to stick out or your pelvis to
   dip, you should be straight up and down.

Watchpoints

- Make sure that the knee goes directly over the
  centre of the foot.
- Do not allow your foot or ankle to roll inwards
  as you bend the knee.
- Keep the pelvis level, both sides of the
  waist long.

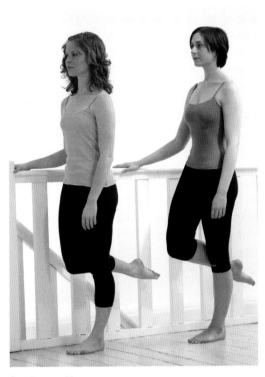

Starting position

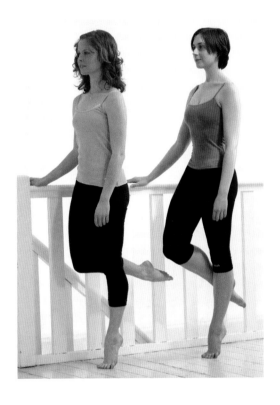

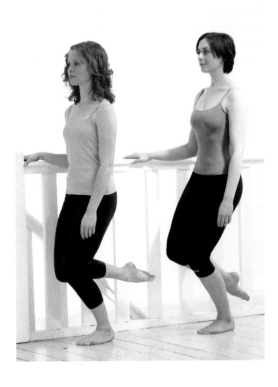

Leg Push Away (*intermediate*)

Enjoy the effect this has on your bottom – it really tones it up. Practise this exercise without weights first. Then slowly build up to weights of 1 kilo each.

Aim

To strengthen the legs and buttocks while keeping a stable core.

Equipment

Leg weights (optional).
A flat pillow (optional).

Starting Position

Lie on your side in a straight line, keeping the natural curves of your back and with a neutral pelvis. Place hip over hip, shoulder over shoulder. Have your underneath arm stretched out under your head in a line with your body. You may like to place a flat pillow between the arm and your head to keep your neck in line. Bend the bottom leg so that it is just less than 90˚ to the body; the knee is also at 90˚. Bring your top arm in front of you in a line with your shoulders; this arm will help to stabilize the upper body as you move. Make sure that the shoulder blade stays down and no tension creeps in.

Action

1   Breathe in wide and full to prepare and lengthen through the spine.
2   Breathe out and zip up and hollow. Stay zipped throughout, and straighten the top leg so that it is in a line with your body and is on a level with your top hip.
3   Breathe in and point the toe. Bend the leg, bringing the knee towards you, still keeping it at hip height.
4   Breathe out and flex the toes towards you. Push the leg away, keeping it at hip height and in a line with your body. Keep good alignment throughout the body.
5   Breathe in and point and bend the leg again.
6   Repeat up to ten times on both sides.

Watchpoints

- Keep the waist lengthened and lifted – do not allow it to sink into the floor.
- Keep checking that the leg is not too high or too low – it should be in a line with your top hip.
- Keep zipping throughout.
- If you are not using weights you might like to imagine that you are pushing your leg through thick treacle (it makes you work harder).

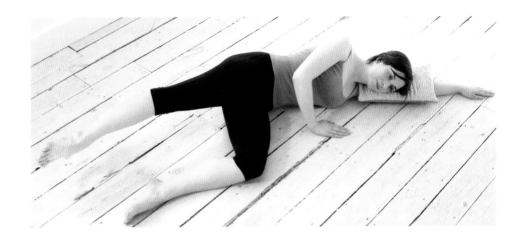

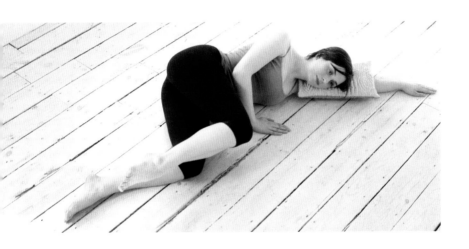

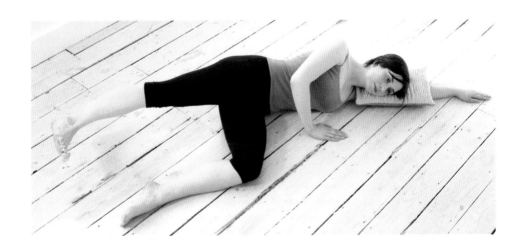

Bridging (*intermediate*)

We have given you two levels for this exercise. Both versions require good core strength. You will feel the work in the supporting buttock.

Aim

To learn lumbar and pelvic stability and to strengthen the buttocks.

Starting Position

Lie in the Relaxation Position (see page 14), but this time have your feet and knees together.

Action

1 Breathe in wide and full to prepare.
2 Breathe out, zip up and hollow, and slowly lift your lower body from the floor. Now, check that you have not arched your back, it should still maintain its natural curves. Place your hands on your pelvis – this is to check that the pelvis stays stable as the legs move.
3 On your next out breath, still zipping and hollowing, straighten one leg, keeping the knees together so that the leg extends in a straight line. Keep your pelvis completely still – do not allow it to dip on one side. Think of keeping both sides of your waist long.
4 Breathe in and bend the knee, returning the foot to the floor.
5 Work up to repeating the exercise five times with each leg before lowering your body back down to the floor.

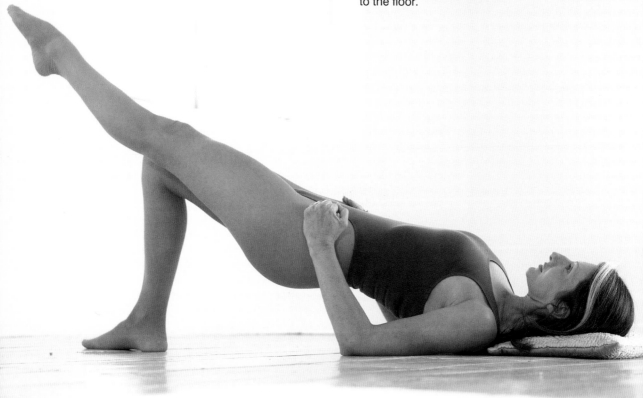

Watchpoints

- When there is a muscle imbalance in the torso there is sometimes a tendency for one side to dominate. As you lift and lower the spine think of a jet taking off and landing right down the central strip of the runway. No high crosswind!
- Keep checking constantly that, as you extend your leg, your pelvis stays in neutral and doesn't dip.
- Use your hands to check for movement in the pelvis; they will also automatically help to keep you a little more stable.

Once you have mastered the first level you can move on to this more advanced level.

Moving on . . .

Action

1 Follow action points 1–3 above, but have your arms down by your sides. Take a breath in and stay zipped throughout. As you breathe out raise the extended leg towards the ceiling, keeping the pelvis still and level.
2 Breathe in and then fold the knee in towards the chest, and breathe out as you lower it back to the starting position.

bottom

Eating to Fight Fat

What you eat is important to the way your body looks. It's unfortunate that the food and drink we enjoy such as alcohol, processed meals and high-fat, salty snacks can encourage fat to be stored around the bottom as well as on the hips and thighs. Dieting – spurred on by celebrity endorsed fads – has become a global obsession. But deprived of our favourite foods and instant results, it's no surprise that we fall back into bad eating habits.

Muscle has a high metabolic so it burns calories quickly. The rest of your body tissue is fat, which does not need oxygen, does not repair itself, and has a low metabolic rate and so it doesn't burn calories. If you want to streamline your body permanently, improve your hair, skin and bones, boost your immune system, improve your energy levels and achieve optimum health, you need to increase your lean body mass (LBM) through correct diet and the right exercise – Pilates plus aerobic activity. Ideally, 90 per cent LBM to 10 per cent fat is right for men; 80–85 per cent LBM to 15–20 per cent fat is right for women.

In addition to the advice given on page 116, try the following:

- Drink at least two litres of still water (mineral or filtered) every day to flush out toxins, assist digestion and keep the body balanced. Drunk either warm or at room temperature, it's a great way to cleanse your body internally and will help to curb your appetite. (A good way to check if you are drinking enough water is to look at the colour of your urine – the clearer your pee, the healthier you'll be!)
- Eat a wide selection of fresh fruit and vegetables – at least five portions during the day. Where possible buy organic and try not to prepare fruit and vegetables too far in advance because they lose nutrients. If they are organic eat the skins as well. If you have to peel them do so thinly as valuable vitamins lie close to the skin.
- Limit your fat intake to between 30 and 35 per cent of your total daily intake of calories. For a woman eating around 2000 calories a day, this equates to around 70 grams.

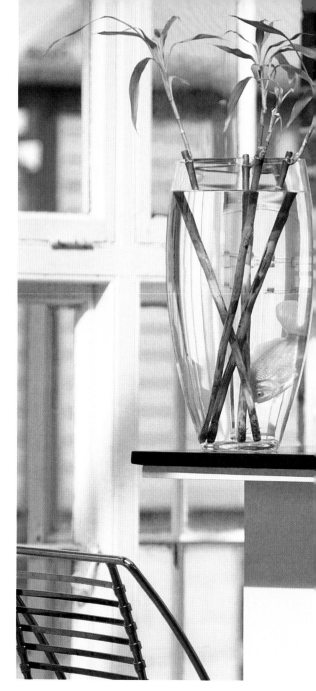

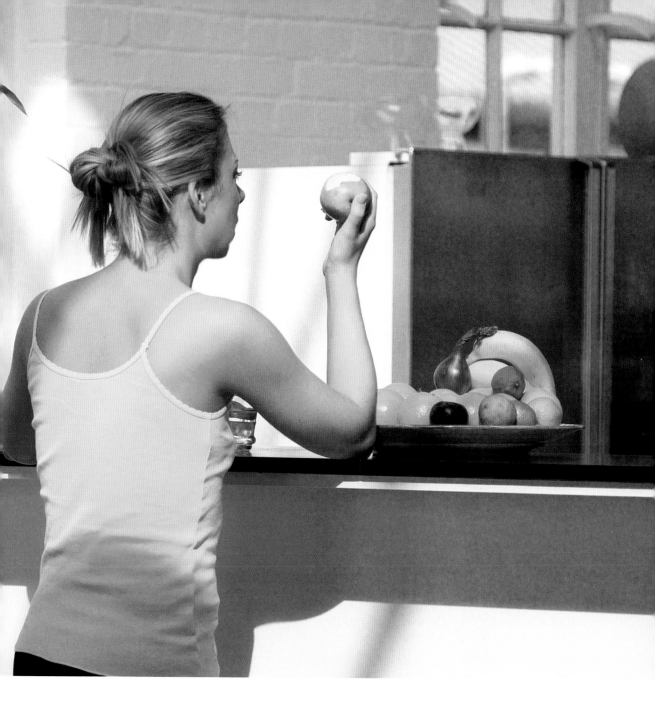

- Replace high-fat and high-sugar snacks such as crisps or chocolate bars with dried fruit, seeds and nuts. These are all rich in vitamins and minerals which are essential if the body is to function at its optimum level.
- When cooking, steam and grill wherever possible instead of frying or boiling. More of the flavour will stay intact and you won't rob the food of its valuable vitamins and minerals.

- Most of all enjoy what you eat. Studies show that the more we enjoy our food, the more nutrients we will absorb from it. If you occasionally give in to a delicious dessert or a take-away pizza, just use common sense and go for the healthiest option (a summer pudding with lots of fruit or a pizza topped with plenty of fresh vegetables, for example).

bottom

Foods to Stock Up On

- Dark green, leafy vegetables such as broccoli and spinach, plus red and orange fruits and vegetables including pumpkins, mangos, apricots and oranges: packed with protective vitamins, minerals and phytochemicals which counteract the damaging effects of free radicals.
- Fennel, cucumber, asparagus and melon: have a mild diuretic effect that helps reduce water retention by flushing out excess fluids.
- Wholewheat bread or pasta and brown rice: contain more fibre, vitamins and minerals than their white equivalents, and help keep the digestive system in good working order.
- Lentils, chickpeas and other pulses: high in fibre, high in protein and low in fat. These foods reduce high cholesterol levels and keep blood-sugar levels stable. They also provide good amounts of iron, essential for healthy blood.
- Seeds (pumpkin, linseed, sesame and sunflower) and oily fish (tuna, salmon, mackerel): rich in essential fatty acids (EFAs) which protect cells in the body from damage. The beneficial oils in these seeds and fish also help regulate the hormones and keep skin supple.

Foods and Drinks to Avoid

- Caffeinated, carbonated or alcohol-based drinks flood the body with toxins and sugar.
- Salt and salty food encourage fluid retention and bloating as well as contributing to heart disease, high blood pressure and osteoporosis.
- Cakes, biscuits and sweets giving a fast sugar fix rather than maintaining a constant sugar levels, encouraging energy dips and cravings.
- Full-fat diary products: choosing reduced-fat alternatives and skimmed milk will significantly reduce your fat intake while ensuring that you still reap the benefits of dairy food's high calcium quota.

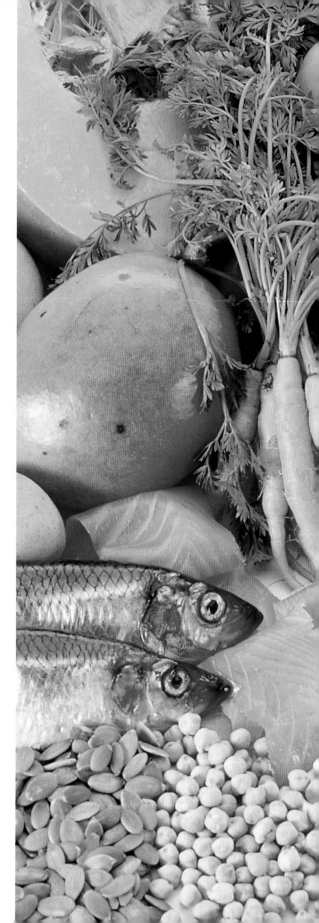

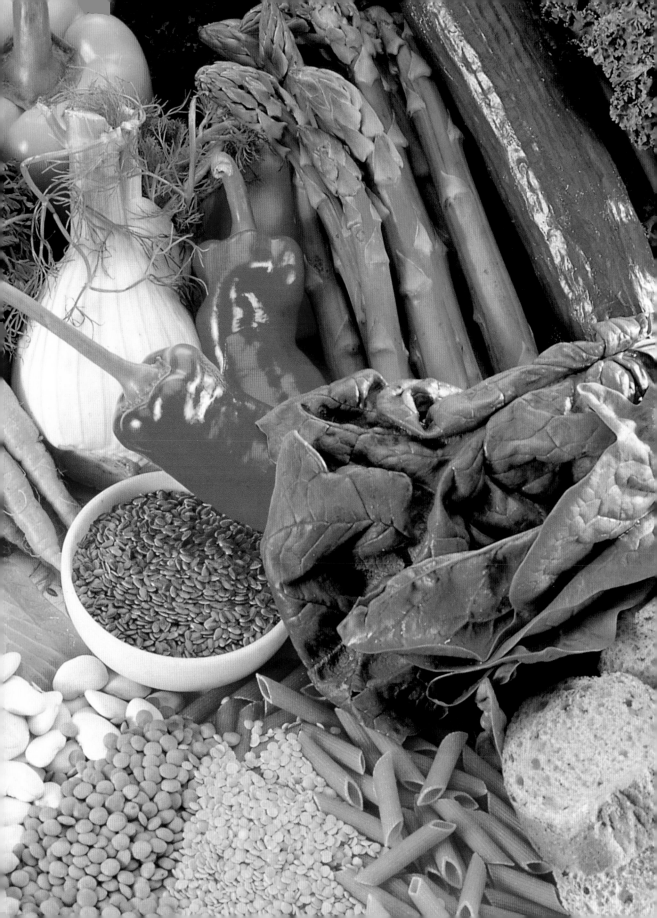

Swordfish with Mango Salsa

Preparation time: **1 hour marinating plus 10 minutes**
Cooking time: **10 minutes**
Serves: **2**

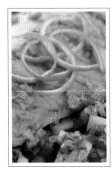

for the fish

2 swordfish steaks

3 tbsp light soy sauce

5cm piece fresh root ginger, finely chopped

2 cloves garlic, crushed or finely chopped

for the salsa

1 ripe mango, peeled and diced

4 plum tomatoes, de-seeded and diced

1 small red onion, finely chopped

4 level tbsp fresh coriander chopped

1 red chilli, de-seeded and finely chopped (optional)

juice of 1 lime

salt and ground black pepper

1 tbsp olive oil

lime zest to garnish

Place the fish in a shallow dish. Mix together the soy sauce, ginger and garlic, then pour over the fish. Cover and place in the fridge for 1 hour.

Mix together all the ingredients for the salsa, cover and chill.

Remove the fish from the marinade and place under a moderately hot grill or put it on a lightly oiled griddle pan. Cook for 4–6 minutes on each side or until cooked through.

Spoon the salsa on to a serving plate, place the swordfish on top, garnish with lime zest and serve immediately.

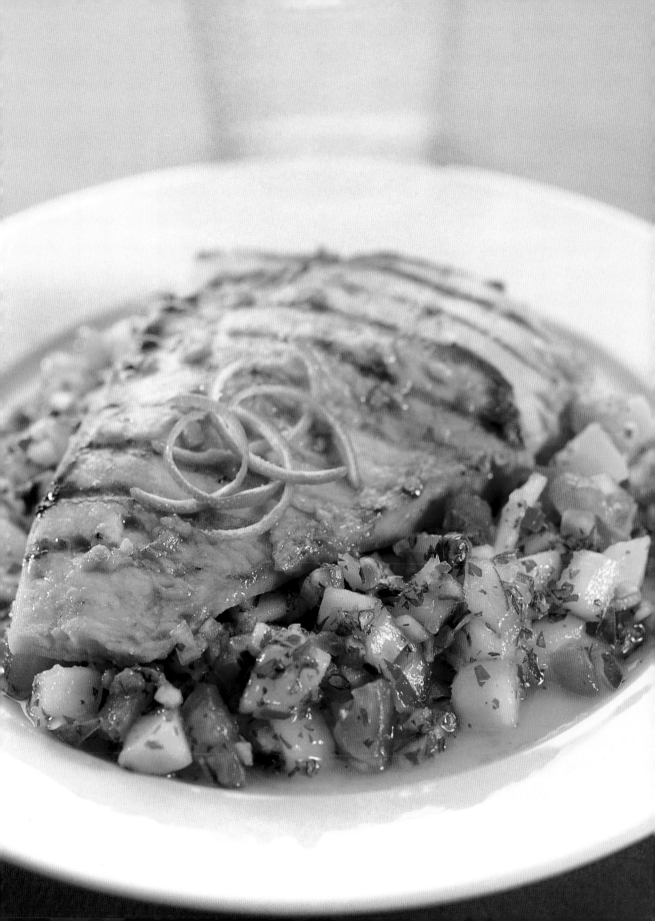

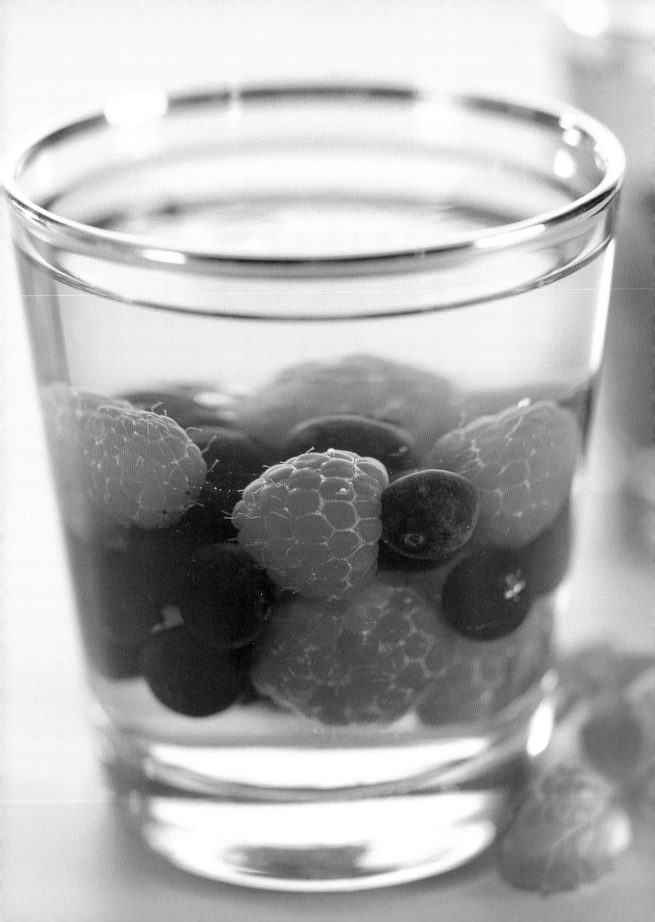

Elderflower Jelly with Raspberries and Blueberries

Preparation time: **5–10 minutes, plus about 3½ hours chilling**
Cooking time: **nil**
Serves: **4**

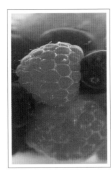

6 tbsp elderflower cordial

1 pint cold water

3 leaves gelatin or vegetarian equivalent

100g raspberries

100g blueberries

Mix the elderflower cordial with the cold water. Place 4 tbsp of the cordial in a heatproof bowl, add the gelatin and leave it to soak for 5 minutes. Place the bowl over a pan of simmering water and stir until the gelatin has dissolved. Stir the mixture into the remaining elderflower cordial.

Divide the fruit between 4 glasses, pour in enough of the liquid to just cover the fruit, then chill for about 30 minutes or until set.

Pour on the remaining liquid and chill for another 3 hours or until set.

If the remaining mixture sets before the final step, place it over a pan of gently simmering water until it becomes liquid again.

DIY Body Brushing

With a celebrity following of models, actresses and other people with beautiful bodies, dry-skin brushing or body brushing is an incredibly effective way to help regain and maintain a svelte silhouette. Not only does it stimulate both the circulation of blood and the lymphatic system (responsible for eliminating toxins and waste fluids), but it smoothes and exfoliates the surface of the skin, improving texture and appearance.

To achieve the best results, brush the skin when it is dry using a natural fibre body brush – choose one with firm bristles that fits comfortably in the palm of your hand. If the sensation of brushing feels uncomfortable at first, use light strokes and increase the pressure over the first week.

The golden rule is to always stroke towards the heart, encouraging rather than fighting the flow of the body's natural systems. Although the contouring effects may take up to three months to see, discipline yourself to do this quick routine first thing every morning and you'll instantly notice an energy boost that helps kick-start your day.

- Making sure you are steady, brush the sole of each foot in turn.
- Work up the lower legs, then from knee to pelvic bone using long, sweeping movements. With each stroke, use your free hand to follow the brush, soothing the skin.
- Continue over the buttocks and hips, then switch to circular, clockwise strokes over the stomach.
- Move on to the arms, starting at the fingertips and sweeping towards the chest, along the shoulders and down the breastbone to the heart.
- Reach round to your back and stroke down each side. If you can reach (or your brush has a long handle attachment), include the middle of the back too.

Contouring Massage for Cellulite

The evolution of what the beauty industry ambitiously first called anti-cellulite cream has been fast and furious. Approaching the new millennium, they conceded that there was more to banishing bumps than applying a product that worked primarily on the epidermis – the skin's outermost layer. Modern formulations, renamed 'firming treatments', offer a more holistic approach to more achievable ends. The instructions that accompany most reputable brands explain that regular exercise and a healthy, balanced diet play an essential role in sculpting your figure.

Firming gels, lotions and creams can work to improve the texture and elasticity of the skin as well as helping to block the ability of cells in the body to store fat. However, their efficacy is greatly increased by massage. This not only helps eliminate water retention and flush out trapped toxins, but also ensures that the treatment you apply is worked deeper into the skin, reaching its target faster. Apply your firming treatment over the buttocks, thighs and stomach after a warm bath or shower, then use these draining massage techniques to speed improvement:

- *Pinching:* Starting above the knee, briskly pinch the fleshy parts of your leg between your thumb and forefingers. Work up the front of each leg, followed by the outside, inside and finally all the way up to the small of the back including the buttocks.
- *Kneading:* Make a fist and use your knuckles to knead the same areas, twisting your hand as you push it into the skin.
- *Stroking:* Using the palms of your hands, finish by firmly stroking the skin five or six times with firm, upwards movements.

For more advice on combating cellulite, turn to Sensational Legs, Spa Style on page 170.

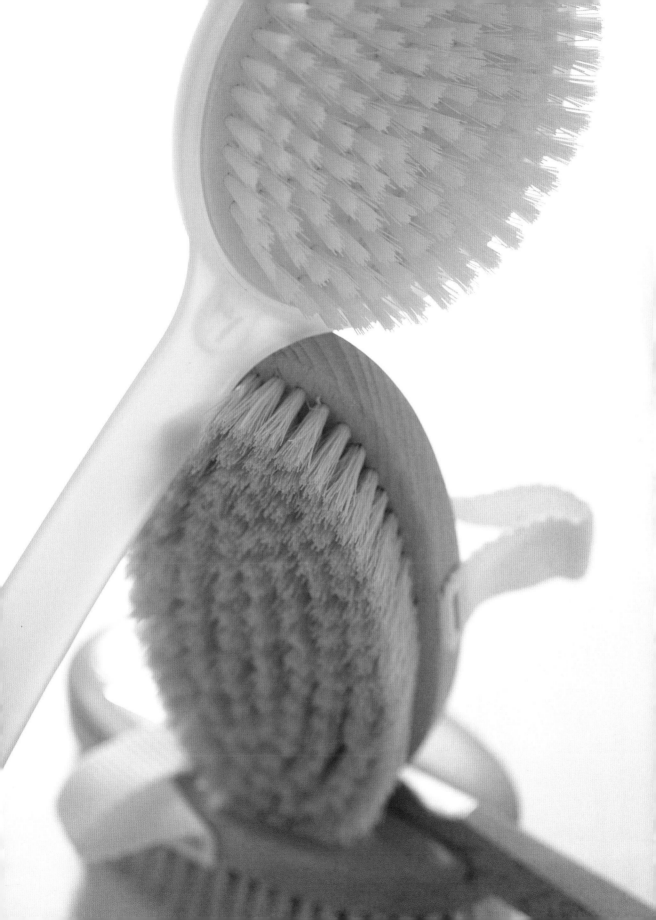

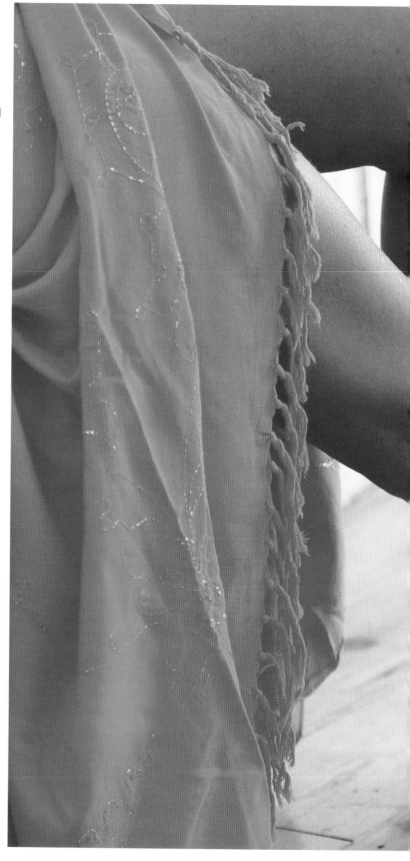

S LEEK, SMOOTH legs are high on most women's wish list. Whether your goal is sculpted calves or firmer thighs, there's a Pilates exercise to help you achieve it. Complemented by an occasional pampering to combat puffiness and the removal of unwanted hair, who says you can't get what you wish for?

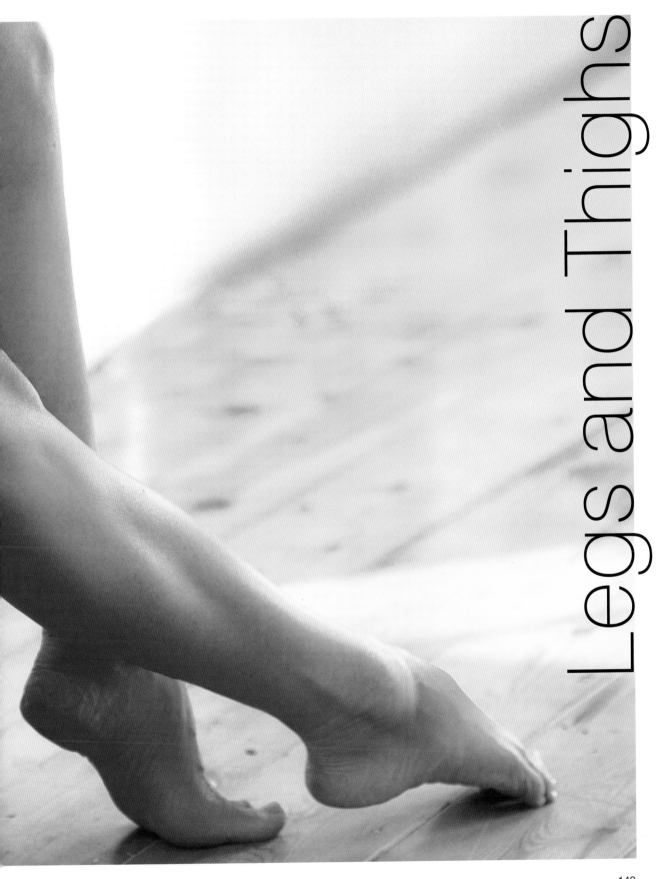

Legs and Thighs

Exercises for the Legs

Sorry, but no amount of exercise will make short legs longer. However, there is plenty you can do to change the shape of your legs: you can add more bulk to your calves which will make your ankles look slimmer; you can tone your thighs, inside and out; you can target the muscles around the knee. But at the same time you must bear in mind the correct balance of the leg muscles. It's no good having super-strong fronts to your thighs without an appropriate amount of strength in the muscles at the back. You must also bear in mind the flexibility of these muscles. Tight hamstrings will pull your pelvis backwards and thus affect the natural curve of your spine. Tight hip flexors particularly rectus femoris – one of your quadriceps – will tilt your pelvis forward increasing the curve of your spine and possibly stressing the lumbar spine. Sometimes, flabby outer and inner thighs relate to an imbalance of muscles and a misalignment of the hip joint.

The key to beautiful legs lies in achieving the right balance in all the muscle groups and in getting the alignment of the feet, knees and hips correct. This is where Pilates comes into its own. By constantly reminding you in the exercises to position your feet, knees and hips carefully we are subtly realigning your legs. Notice the directions in Standing Correctly (see page 6). Whenever you are asked to bend the knees, it is always so that the knee passes over the second toe, for example in the Barre Exercise on page 152. This attention to detail ensures that you are working the legs in a balanced way and it will ultimately affect their whole shape. We may not be able to promise you Darcey Bussell's legs, but we can offer you the best you can naturally achieve.

Hamstring Strengthener/ Stretch (*beginners*)

With this exercise you first work the hamstring muscles (which run along the backs of your thighs) and then you stretch them.

Aim
To stretch and strengthen the hamstrings.

Equipment
A towel (optional).
A flat, firm pillow (optional).

Starting Position
Lie in the Relaxation Position (see page 14). Check that your pelvis is in neutral – it must stay in neutral throughout. Bring one knee towards your chest and clasp it behind the thigh; if you cannot reach comfortably then wrap the towel around the back of the thigh. Hold the towel from underneath with your palms towards you.

Action
1 Breathe in wide and full to prepare.
2 Breathe out and zip up and hollow. Stay zipped throughout, and slowly push into your hands or the towel. Breathe normally as you count to six. Make sure that your back does not arch and that you do not strain. Your upper body should stay relaxed and open.
3 After six seconds, breathe in and then out as you slowly straighten the leg into the air. Your tailbone stays down on the mat. Try to relax the muscles around the front of the hip.
4 Breathing normally now, hold the stretch for the count of twenty seconds, or until you feel the muscle release.
5 Relax the leg by gently bending it again.
6 Repeat twice to each leg.

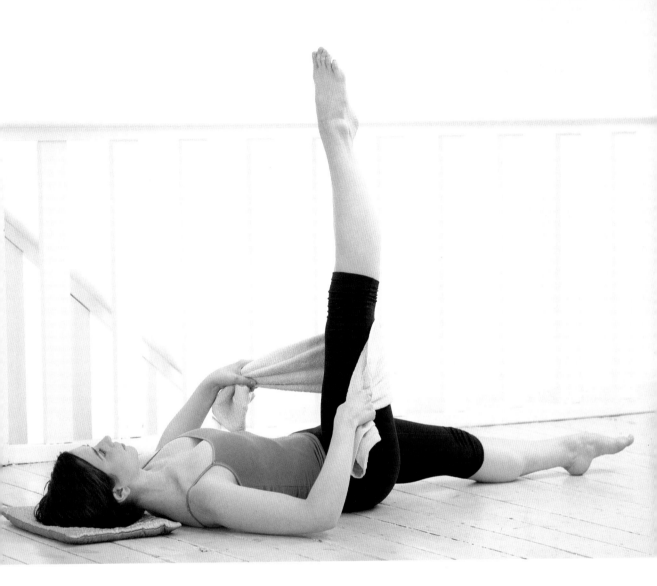

Watchpoints

- Don't allow the pelvis to twist as you straighten the leg. Anchoring navel to spine will help you: north to south, east to west.
- Keep your tailbone down as you stretch the leg.
- Check your neck. Often the neck shortens and arches back as the hamstrings are stretched. If this happens, place a small flat firm pillow under your head to keep the neck long. Think of softening the neck and breastbone and of opening the elbows.
- Don't strain – ease the leg out, gently stretching it within your limits.
- Keep breathing while you push against your hand or towel.

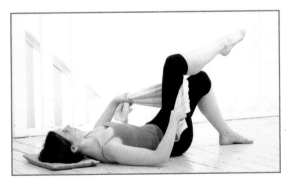

Starting position

legs and thighs

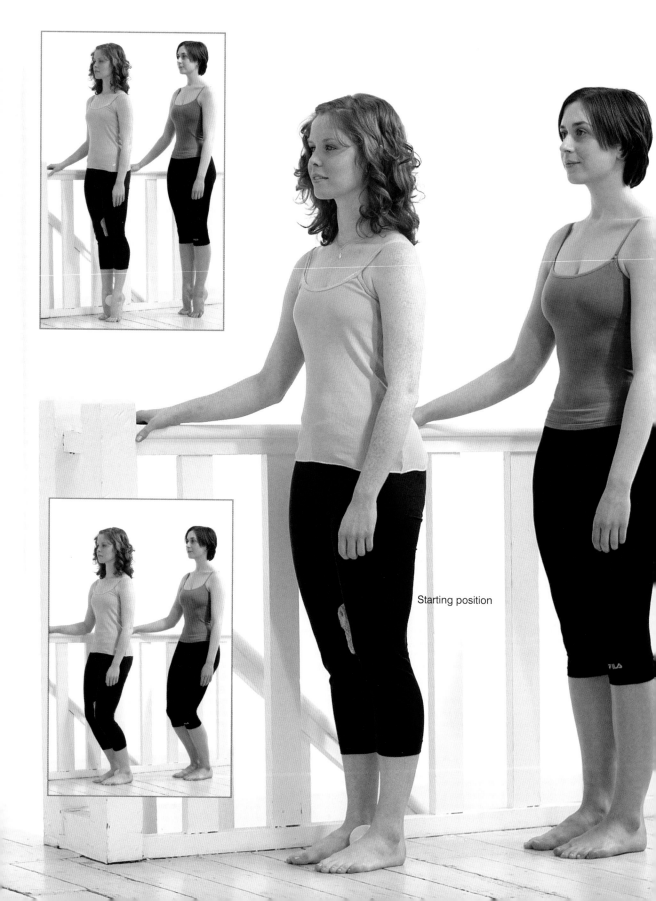

Starting position

Up and Down Barre Exercise (*beginners*)

Alignment is everything for this exercise. By correctly bending the knees over the feet and keeping them centrally over the second toes, you are working the thigh muscles as nature intended. Deviate just a little and you have the potential for an imbalance which, if it becomes habitual, could lead to knee problems.

The group of muscles known collectively as the quadriceps is, as one would expect from the name, made up of four muscles. If one of these four becomes dominant, the delicate balance is upset and the knee joint is compromised.

The muscle most likely to weaken is vastus medialis, the main stabilizer of the knee joint. It has its own blood supply and begins to waste after just twenty-four hours of bed rest!

This is also an excellent exercise to do if you're on a long flight as it activates the deep calf pump and boosts circulation in the legs.

Aim

To strengthen the leg muscles, especially the vastus medialis, and improve leg circulation. To help learn good body alignment.

Equipment

Two tennis balls or one tennis ball and a small pillow.

Starting Position

Stand sideways on to a wall and place the tennis ball between your ankles, just below the inside ankle bone. Place another tennis ball or a small pillow between the thighs just above the knees. Remind yourself of all the directions given in Standing Correctly on page 6. Hold onto the wall.

Action

1 Breathe in and lengthen up through the spine – imagine someone is pulling you up from the top of your head, but that there is also a weight on your tailbone, anchoring your spine.
2 Breathe out, zip up and hollow, and rise up on your toes.
3 Breathe in.
4 Breathe out, and slowly lengthen your heels back down on the floor away from the top of your head. Imagine that your head stays up.
5 When your heels are on the floor, slightly bend your knees directly over your feet, keeping the heels down. Do not allow your bottom to stick out.
6 Repeat ten times.

Watchpoints

- Do not allow your bottom to stick out as you bend the knees.
- Keep the heels on the ground as you bend the knees.
- Keep the weight evenly balanced on the feet.
- Keep lengthening upwards throughout.
- Try not to tip forward or back – straight up and down.

Side-lying Leg Circles (*intermediate*)

Another wonderful exercise to tone and shape the upper leg. It also works the core trunk muscles.

Aim
To strengthen the upper legs and buttock muscles.

Equipment
A flat pillow (optional).

Starting Position
Lie on your side in a straight line keeping the natural curves of your back and a neutral pelvis. Place hip over hip, shoulder over shoulder. Have your underneath arm stretched out under your head in a line with your body (you may like to place a flat pillow between the arm and your head to keep your neck in line). Bend the bottom leg so that it is just less than 90° to the body; the knee is also at 90°. Bring your top arm in front of you in a line with your shoulders. This arm will help to stabilize the upper body as you move. Make sure that the shoulder blade stays down and that no tension creeps in.

Action
1. Breathe in wide and full to prepare and lengthen through the body.
2. Breathe out and zip up and hollow. Stay zipped throughout, and slowly straighten the top leg so that it is in a line with your body and at the same height as your top hip.
3. Point the toes.
4. Breathe in and slowly draw five small circles (about the size of a grapefruit) with the whole leg, the action originating in the hip joint. Keep lengthening through the leg the whole time.
5. Breathe out and draw five circles in the other direction.
6. Repeat four sets of five circles before replacing the leg on the bent underneath leg. Then turn over and repeat with the other leg.

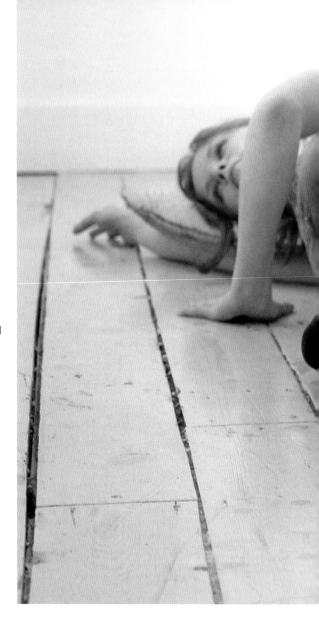

Watchpoints
- Keep the waist lengthened and lifted – do not allow it to sink into the floor.
- Keep checking that the leg is not too high or too low – it should be in a line with your top hip.
- Keep zipping throughout.

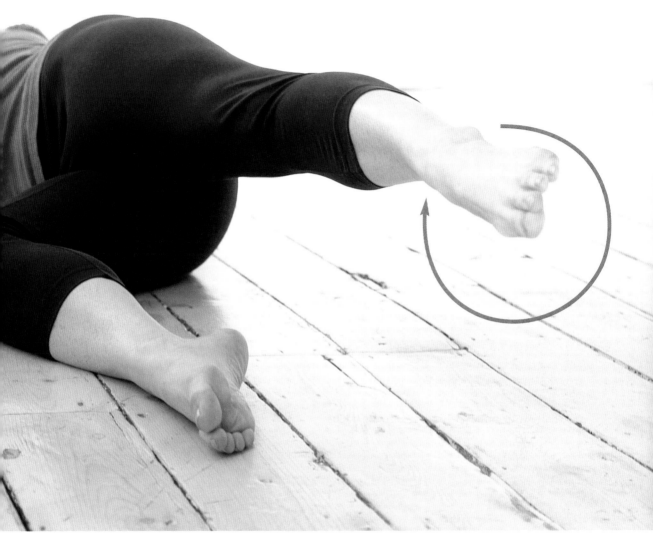

Moving on . . .

If you want to challenge your core stability a little more then stretch out the bottom leg so that it is at a slight angle in front of you.

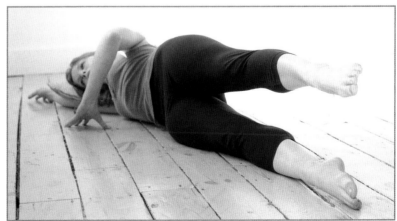

Moving on . . .

Passé Développés (*intermediate*)

You can see the ballet influence in this exercise. It really targets the upper thigh and deep buttock muscles – think of dancers' long never-ending legs.

Aim
To achieve the correct balance in the leg, and hip and buttock muscles. To achieve control of the muscles around the hip joint.

Equipment
A foam triangular cushion or a couple of large pillows.
Leg weights of ½–1 kilo each weight.

Action
1   Remember the exercise Turning Out the Leg in Pelvic Stability on page 23. You are going to do the same action now, turning out the leg from the hip without losing the stability of the pelvis.
2   Breathe in to prepare.
3   Breathe out, zip up and hollow, and fold your knee up. Turn it out from the hip, without moving the pelvis.
4   Breathe in, still zipped and hollowed, and slowly straighten the leg, keeping it turned out from the hip and in a line with it. Keep your tailbone on the floor.

Starting Position
Lie on the cushion or the pillows. The idea is that your upper back is supported, but that your lower ribcage, waist and pelvis are on the mat. Your knees are bent, hip-width apart and parallel.

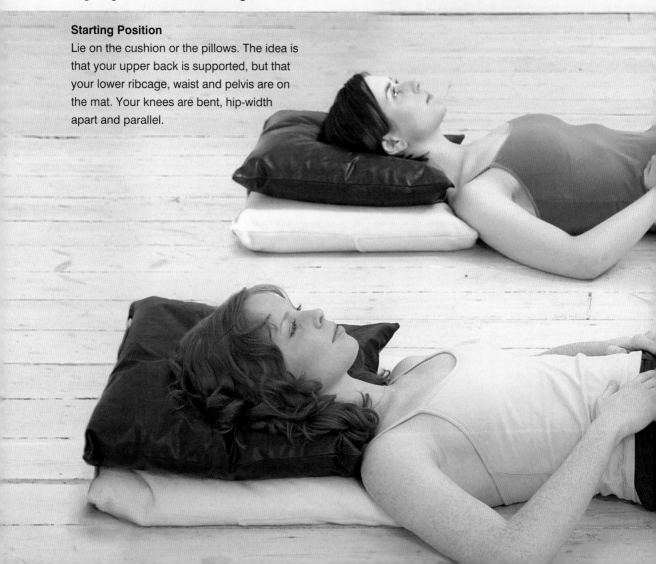

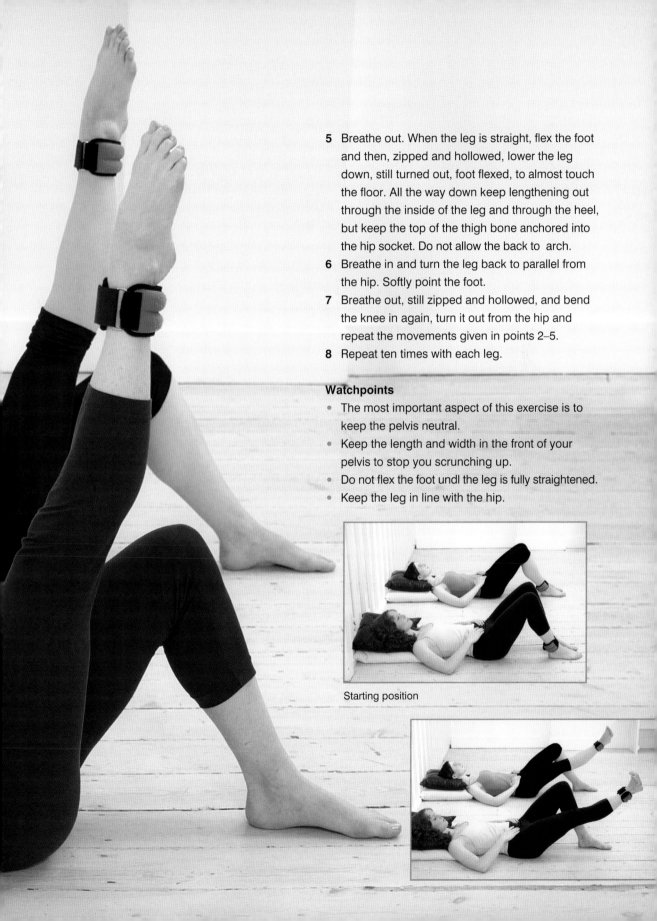

5 Breathe out. When the leg is straight, flex the foot and then, zipped and hollowed, lower the leg down, still turned out, foot flexed, to almost touch the floor. All the way down keep lengthening out through the inside of the leg and through the heel, but keep the top of the thigh bone anchored into the hip socket. Do not allow the back to arch.

6 Breathe in and turn the leg back to parallel from the hip. Softly point the foot.

7 Breathe out, still zipped and hollowed, and bend the knee in again, turn it out from the hip and repeat the movements given in points 2–5.

8 Repeat ten times with each leg.

Watchpoints

- The most important aspect of this exercise is to keep the pelvis neutral.
- Keep the length and width in the front of your pelvis to stop you scrunching up.
- Do not flex the foot undl the leg is fully straightened.
- Keep the leg in line with the hip.

Starting position

Side-lying Quadriceps Stretch (*beginners*)

We have included a lot of thigh-strengthening exercises, but it is equally important that these muscles maintain good length and flexibility.

Aim

To stretch out the quadricep muscles which run along the front of the thigh and the hip flexors. To lengthen and iron out the front of the body, especially around the front of the hips which can get very tight if you sit all day. To maintain good alignment of the torso by using the waist muscles and the shoulder stabilizers.

Notice the position of the pelvis. We ask you to tuck it under slightly, that is tilt it backwards (to north) losing neutral. No, we haven't gone crazy but there is a danger with this exercise that you may arch the back and stress the lumbar spine – so it is better to play safe and tuck under slightly. Also, by tilting the pelvis you can isolate the hip flexor muscles.

Equipment

A scarf (optional).
A flat pillow (optional).

Starting Position

Lie on your side, your head resting on your extended arm (you may like a flat pillow between the head and the arm to keep the neck in line). Have the knees curled up at slightly less than 90° to your body. Your back should be in a straight line, but with its natural curves. Line up all your bones on top of each other – foot over foot, knee over knee, hip over hip and shoulder over shoulder.

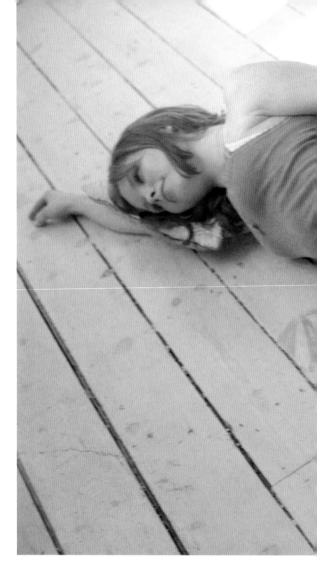

Action

1 Breathe in wide and full to prepare and lengthen through the spine.

2 Breathe out, zip up and hollow, and bend the top knee towards you taking hold of the front of the foot if you can reach it (you may need to use a scarf).

3 Breathe in and check your pelvic position. You would normally be in neutral in this position but this time you may tuck your pelvis under (see Aim).

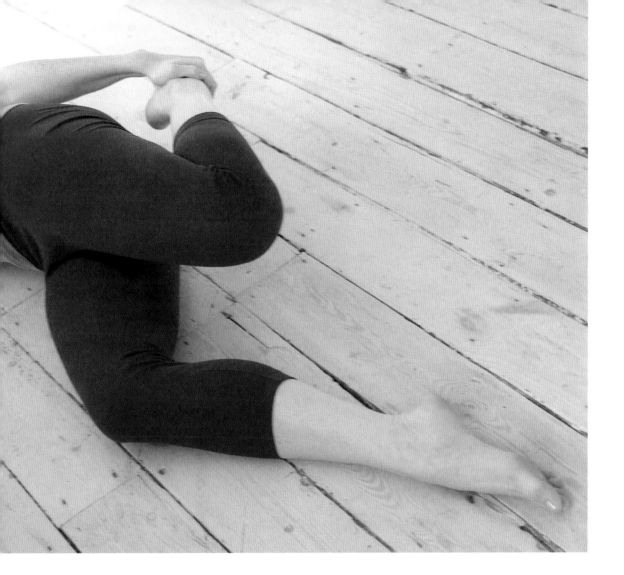

4 Breathe out and zip up and hollow. Stay zipped throughout, and gently take the leg behind you to stretch the front of the thigh. Do not arch the back, keep the tailbone lengthening away from the top of your head.

5 Hold the stretch for about twenty seconds or until you feel the muscle release, working the waist the whole time and keeping the length in the trunk.

6 After twenty seconds slowly relax the stretch by bringing the leg back in front of you, zipping throughout.

7 Repeat twice on each side.

Watchpoints

- Keep the shoulder blades down into the back and the gap between the arms and the shoulders.
- Do not collapse forward. Keep the upper body open, and the waist long.
- If you cannot reach the foot or the knee feels stressed, use the scarf wrapped over the front of the foot.

> **Warning:** please take advice if you have a knee injury. You may need to use a scarf to hook over the foot so that there is less pressure on the knee, or you may need to leave this one out.

TFL Stretch (*intermediate*)

There is a band of muscles which runs along the side of the thighs and these can become very tight. They are notoriously difficult to stretch and you often need a good massage to soften them. It's probably worth spending a few minutes kneading them before you try this stretch. If you do, work upwards from just above the side of the knee to the hip.

Aim

To stretch the thigh muscles.

Equipment

A scarf (optional).
A flat pillow.

Starting Position

As for the Side-lying Quadriceps Stretch (see pages 158). In fact it's a good idea to do this exercise straight afterwards.

Action

1 Follow Action points 1–5 for the Side-lying Quadriceps Stretch on pages 158–9, then bring your bottom foot up and hook it over the top leg just above the knee.
2 It is crucial that you do not tilt the pelvis at this point; the waist stays long and in neutral. The pelvis stays square.
3 Breathe normally as you stretch for about thirty seconds or until you feel the muscle release.
4 Then slowly release by bringing the leg back in front of you.
5 Repeat twice on each side.

Warning: avoid this exercise if you have knee problems. It often feels a little uncomfortable around the knee as you do it, but it should not hurt.

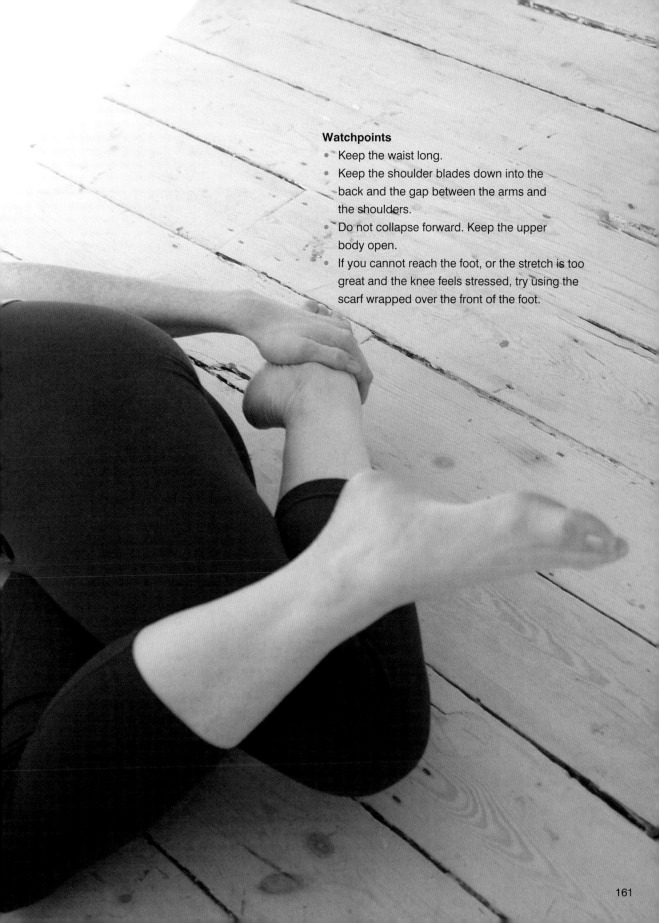

Watchpoints

- Keep the waist long.
- Keep the shoulder blades down into the back and the gap between the arms and the shoulders.
- Do not collapse forward. Keep the upper body open.
- If you cannot reach the foot, or the stretch is too great and the knee feels stressed, try using the scarf wrapped over the front of the foot.

Legs up the Wall

This series of wall stretches looks deceptively easy. They require you to have your legs up a wall – a fabulous position for improving their circulation. Elevated, the calf pump works doubly well. As the muscles tighten and relax, they help the veins to pump the blood back to the heart (venous return). If you suffer from varicose veins, where the valves in the veins have failed and blood seeps out into the surrounding tissue, there exists a blockage in the system which these exercises will help to clear.

Aim
As well as relaxing and widening the torso, especially around the shoulder blades, this exercise will lengthen the entire spine. It also improves the circulation in the legs.

Equipment
A flat pillow (optional).

Starting Position for all Wall Exercises
There is no elegant way to get into this position. The easiest way is to roll on to your side, shuffle your bottom up as close to the wall as you can and then swing your legs round and up the wall. (On a practical note, you would be wise not to use a wall covered with your best designer wallpaper, as you are likely to leave heel marks on it!) Have your buttocks as close to the wall as possible. If you have short hamstrings this will prove difficult, so only come as close as is comfortable – your tailbone should still touch the floor. Have the pelvis in neutral and place a flat pillow under your head if necessary. The legs should be straight (if possible) and hip-width apart.

Note: when you have finished all the wall exercises roll on to your side and rest for a few minutes before standing up.

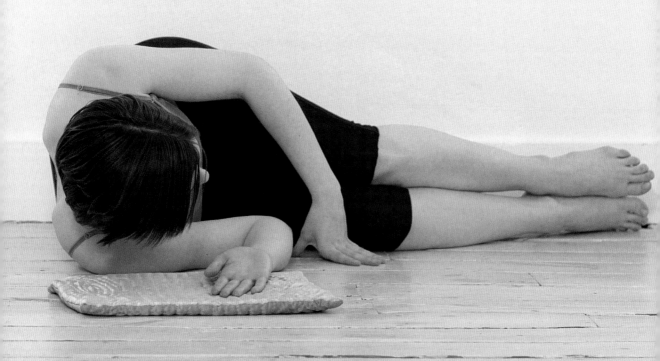

Action

1 Take your arms behind you soft and wide, and relax them onto the floor if you can. If not, leave them down by your sides.

2 Remember to keep your shoulder blades down into your back – do not allow the upper back to arch – and allow the spine to lengthen and the neck to release.

3 Work up to spending three minutes in this position. Bear in mind that if you are going to continue with the following exercises, you will be here for quite some time, so judge it carefully.

4 When you have finished, bend the knees gently and bring your arms down by your sides.

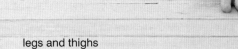

Ankle Circles (*beginners*)

Aim

This exercise will stretch the hamstrings, work the muscles of the lower legs, mobilize and strengthen the ankle joints and improve circulation.

Action

1 Lie with your legs hip-distance apart and parallel.
2 Check that you are square to the wall and not at an angle and that your pelvis is in neutral.
3 Keeping the legs completely still, rotate the feet outwardly, circling from the ankle joints. You should be circling very, very slowly and as far as you can.
4 Repeat ten circles in each direction.

Watchpoints

• Don't just twiddle the toes around, work from the ankle joints.
• Where it says keep the legs still, that means still! And in parallel.

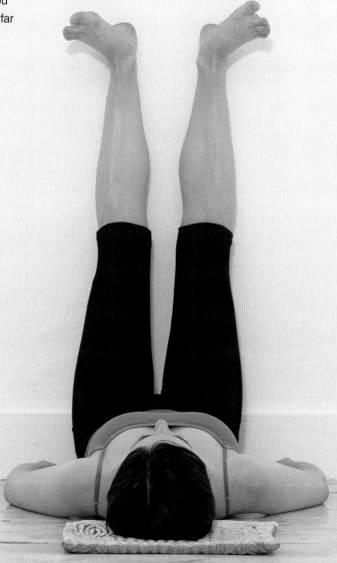

The Wide Leg Stretch (*beginners / intermediate*)

Action

1 Check that you are square on to the wall.
2 If your hamstrings are tight then come away from
   the wall a little. Your tailbone must stay down on
   the floor or you will lose neutral.
3 Slowly lower your legs to the sides until you feel
   a comfortable stretch in the inner thighs. Make
   sure that both legs are at the same height and
   that the pelvis stays level.
4 Relax in this position for a few minutes (not more
   than three), then use your hands to bring your
   legs together.

When you have finished the wall exercises roll
on to your side and rest for a few minutes before
standing up.

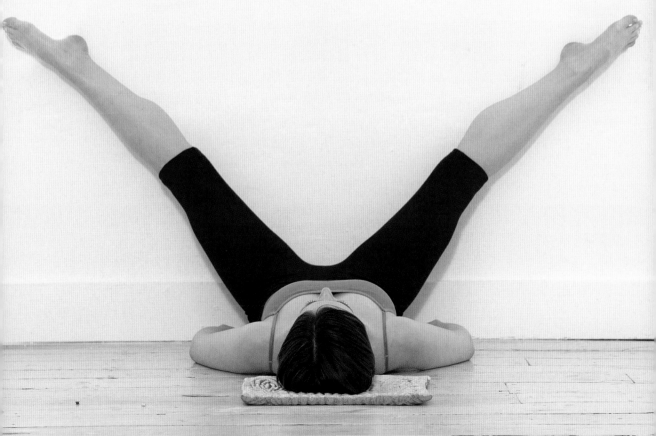

Hair-free How To

From eyebrows to ankles, the search for the perfect hair-removal technique has become something of the Holy Grail of beauty. While where and how much you remove is mainly down to cultural heritage, the methods used are often the same. Decide what's right for you according to where the hair is, how much money you have to spend and how high your pain threshold is.

Shaving

Best for underarms and legs

As the fastest, cheapest and – assuming you are deft with a razor – least painful way to remove hair, shaving is the most popular choice. Choose a razor with a lubricating strip and change the blade after four or five uses to ensure that it glides over the skin without causing nicks or cuts. Also apply a shaving oil, foam or gel to warm, wet skin first and wait thirty seconds while it softens the hair to give a satin-smooth finish. The drawbacks are that re-growth starts to show within two days and can look thicker and darker as the tip of the hair is blunt.

Waxing

Best for legs, arms and bikini line

First-timers should book into a reputable beauty salon, as waxing is a learned skill. If you have the confidence to try it at home once you have watched the professionals at work there are plenty of good DIY kits available. Be warned though – you'll need at least twenty minutes, as well as the ability to handle the agony alone (chatting to a beautician always seems to divert attention from the pain). The benefits are that waxing leaves a clean, smooth finish for at least a week, with hairs often reappearing finer and sparser. Most at-home kits involve applying a thick layer of warm wax to the area, then placing a cotton or linen strip on top before quickly pulling it back as you hold the skin taut. Alternatively, you can try stick-on, pull-off gel patches. As waxing doesn't exfoliate the skin, remember to use a body scrub regularly to prevent ingrowing hairs.

Depilatory creams

Best for underarms, legs and bikini line

Available in a cream or gel formula, these chemical mixtures effectively dissolve the entire hair shaft in as little as five minutes, leaving you hair free for about a week. Simply apply and wait the recommended time before gently buffing off with damp cotton wool or a flannel. Do a patch test twenty-four hours in advance to check for skin irritation though.

Threading

Best for eyebrows and facial hair

This traditional Indian technique has become popular in the West over the last few years, largely due to its celebrity following. A length of specially made cotton thread is held against the skin and twisted so that it grasps individual hairs, allowing them to be pulled out at the root without breaking (a common problem when you use tweezers). The feeling is akin to plucking, but the result is more like waxing – every hair is removed, leaving the skin totally smooth. It's fast, effective and devotees report that hairs grow back finer and slower – the only problem is that you can't do it yourself.

Electrolysis

Best for anywhere on the face, except the eyebrows

Until the arrival of lasers, electrolysis was the only method of hair removal to offer some permanence. It uses an electric current, passed through a needle and down the hair shaft to create a chemical reaction that kills hairs in their growing phase (the other two phases are sleeping and shedding). The needle has to be inserted directly into each hair shaft, making the process potentially slow, painful and with the risk of scarring. If you do want to try electrolysis, choose a newer, non-invasive method such as Transdermal Electrolysis (TE).

Laser Hair Removal

Best for face, bikini line and underarms

Laser hair removal has evolved rapidly since becoming widely available several years ago and now offers successful treatment for most colourings (the exceptions being freckled skin and white hair). Lasers emit wavelengths that are conducted down the hair shaft where they react with the pigment that gives hair its colour, creating enough heat to destroy it at the root. This feels like a hot pinprick and you'll smell burning, but as more than one hair is treated at a time, lasers are fast and effective. Before committing to a course, it is essential to have a patch test done and to talk to the consultant in depth about what will best suit you. Book at least three sessions, six to eight weeks apart – like electrolysis, hair can only be removed permanently during its growing phase. You will also need a 'top up' session about twelve months later to tackle any hair follicles that were previously inactive. Prices vary depending on the laser and the area being treated, but expect to pay a minimum of several hundred pounds.

Pampering Tired Legs

Target swollen legs and aching muscles with these simple techniques, designed to bring relief quickly and easily.

Quick-fix Leg Revivers

Soothe and cool tired legs with one of these instant revitalisers:

Clarins Energizing Emulsion For Tired Legs

Lancôme Aroma Calm Relaxing Leg and Foot Gel

Elemis Musclease Active Body Concentrate

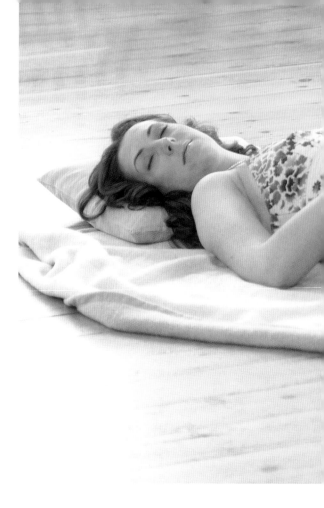

After a Hard Workout

Despite stretching before and afterwards, by the end of a gruelling exercise session muscles often ache. Choose a warming muscle rub or massage oil that will soften and relax tension and use the 'friction' massage technique to increase the effect: taking each leg in turn, place both palms flat behind the knees, then briskly rub up and down for one to two minutes. Repeat on each side and on the front of the legs too.

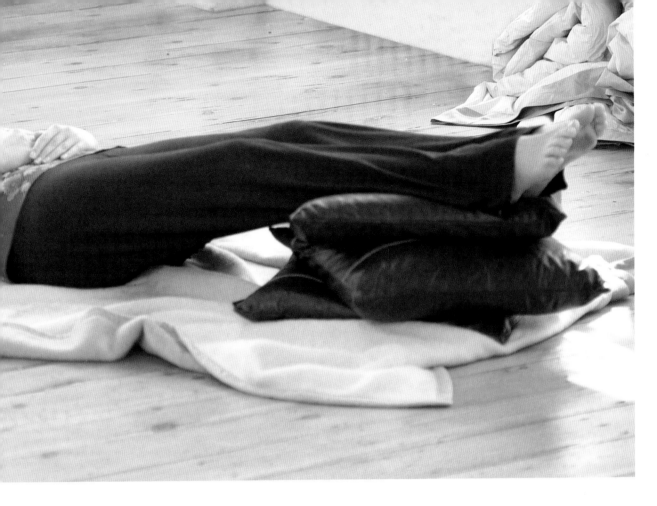

After a Long-haul Flight

The effects on the body of high-altitude travel, combined with sitting in a stationary position for hours, often lead fluid to collect in the ankles causing them to puff up. Although temporary, this swelling can be painful, so move and stretch your legs as much as possible during your journey and after touchdown. As soon as you get time to relax, lie flat and prop up your lower legs on a couple of pillows so they are higher than your head. Spend a few minutes circling your ankles clockwise, then anti-clockwise, to stimulate the blood flow and help drain away excess fluids. Also try the Legs Up the Wall series of exercises on pages 162–5.

After Being on Your Feet All Day

Standing up for long periods, whether for work or pleasure, puts a strain on the leg muscles all the way up to the back. The easiest way to soothe these tired limbs is a fifteen-minute soak in the bath. Fill the tub with warm water and dissolve a handful of mineral-rich, muscle-easing Dead Sea salts under the tap. If you prefer a more fragrant option, add ten to twenty drops of bath oil instead – choose a pre-blended mix that includes essential oils such as rosemary, wintergreen, lavender and juniper.
If you find your ankles or feet are swollen too, try the post-flight technique once you have finished bathing.

Sensational Legs, Spa Style

Top of the list of body bugbears for modern women? Cellulite – believed to be fat and toxins trapped just underneath the surface of the skin. Usually concentrated on the bottom and stomach as well as hips and thighs, this fatty build-up pushes the skin's cells outward, creating the bumpy, uneven surface that's frequently called the orange-peel effect. To contour the legs, combine this daily spa-inspired routine with your Pilates programme and a balanced diet.

- Give your whole body a wake-up call first thing in the morning with two minutes of body brushing. Following the technique on page 146 will help streamline legs by boosting the circulation and lymphatic system, both of which are essential to eliminating excess fluids and toxins from the body.
- In the shower, exfoliation – especially around the ankles and knees where dead skin cells accumulate in flaky patches – will encourage soft, glowing skin. Use a body scrub or mix a handful of sea salt with a few drops of stimulating rosemary or peppermint essential oil.
- If you are in the bath, keep the circulation and lymphatic system invigorated with this popular hydrotherapy technique. Before stepping out, drain the water to calf level, then use a shower attachment to jet cold water slowly over the legs, stomach and buttocks. Switch the shower back to warm for one minute, then to cold again to finish.
- Briskly towel-dry the body before applying a firming body treatment, designed to tone and tighten affected areas. Available as creams, gels, oils and lotions, most modern formulations claim to inhibit the body's ability to store fat, while increasing collagen production in the skin so it becomes more elastic with a smoother, softer texture. If you have a few minutes to spare, turn to page 146 for fantastic contouring massage techniques.

Body-sculpting Bestsellers

Lancôme Aroma Fit Ultra-Slimming Serum

Clarins: Body Lift Contour Control

Yves Saint Laurent Ligne Pure

Christian Dior Body Bikini Minceur Body-Contouring and Refining Essence

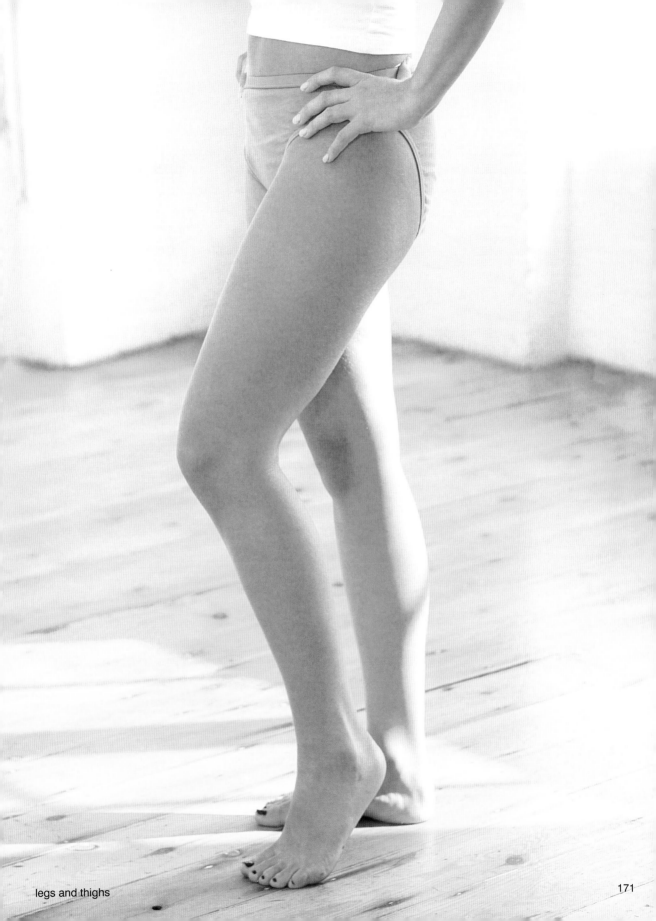

legs and thighs

OFTEN EXPOSED, but usually neglected, hands and feet can reveal our age, reflect our lifestyle and even indicate illness. Regularly lavishing even the smallest amount of attention on them will not only ensure a polished finish to your appearance, but also help relieve mental and muscular tension, increase flexibility and stimulate the circulation.

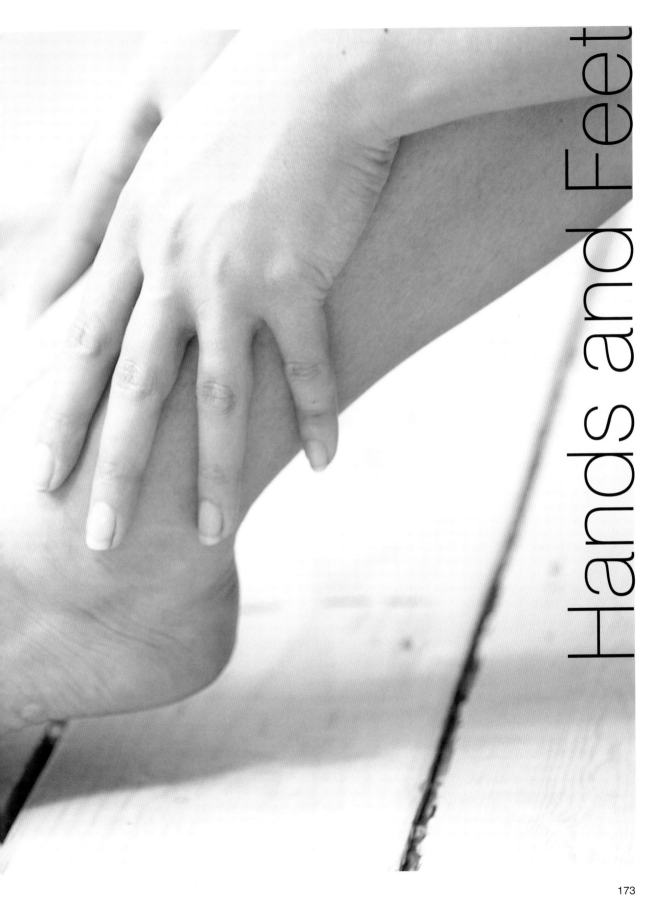

Hands and Feet

Exercises for the Hands

Think for a moment of all the complex and intricate things you can do with your hands. They are amazingly dexterous but also need to be sensitive and strong. The following exercises are great for keeping your hands in good shape. They can be done either sitting or standing tall.

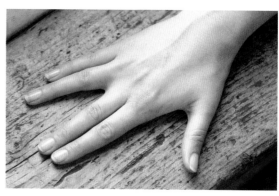
Create a gap in the middle

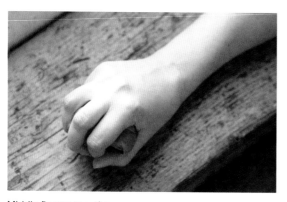
Middle fingers together

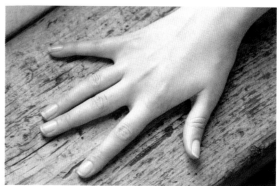
Middle fingers together

Exercise One

Action

1 Sit tall with your hand resting on a table. Stay square to the table.
2 Grip a handful of Play-Doh (or a soft squidgy ball) and squeeze it using all your fingers and your thumb.
3 Hold the squeeze and then release.
4 Repeat ten times with each hand, keeping tension away from your shoulders and neck.

Exercise Two

Action

1 Hold your hands out in front of you, elbows soft.
2 Take the first and second fingers together away from the third and fourth fingers, creating a gap in the middle.
3 Return to centre.
4 Repeat eight times.
6 Then leaving the second and third fingers in the centre, take the first and fourth fingers away.
7 Return to centre.
8 Repeat eight times.

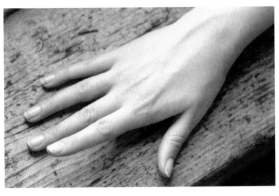

Lift the fingers . . .

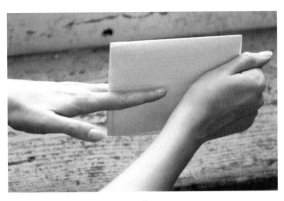

Hold the paper between two fingers

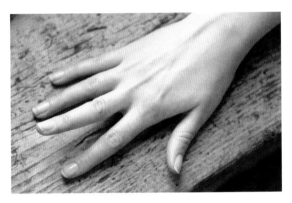

. . . one by one

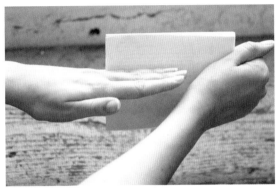

Pull the sheet of paper

Exercise Three – The Mexican Wave

Action

1 Sit tall at a table with your forearms resting on the surface, palms down. Keep your shoulder blades down into your back, neck released, lengthening through the spine.
2 Place your hands flat on the table top.
3 One by one lift the fingers and thumb, trying to keep the others down as you do so.

Exercise Four

This works the deep muscles of the hand.

Action

1 Sitting tall, have your elbows close into your body, shoulder blades down into your back, neck released above.
2 Hold a sheet of paper between two fingers of your left hand. Keep the fingers straight.
3 With your right hand try to pull the sheet from between the fingers; resist with the fingers of your left hand by squeezing them together. Make sure that you continue to breathe normally and do not create extra tension elsewhere in the body.
4 Repeat by putting the sheet between all the fingers of both hands in turn.

DIY Manicure

Your Complete Manicure Kit

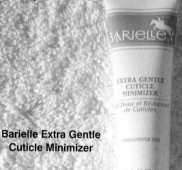

**Barielle Extra Gentle
Cuticle Minimizer**

**Space NK Nail
Polish Remover**

**Barielle Professional
Protective Hand Cream**

Space NK Nail File

SPACE.NK

BARiELLE

PROFESSIONAL
PROTECTIVE
HAND CREAM

Crème Professionnelle
Protectrice Pour
Les Mains

NET WT. 4 OZ. / 113.4g

CLINIQUE

soft polish
body exfoliator

massage douceur
exfoliant corporel

**orange
sticks**

cotton wool

**Clinique Soft Polish
Body Exfoliator**

7 FL.OZ./200ml℮

Manicure Masterclass

Thanks to the elements and dehydrating detergents, hands age faster than any other part of the body. Keep them in peak condition by following this once-a-week, ten-minute manicure.

1 Remove dirt and traces of old nail varnish with a cotton-wool ball soaked in nail polish remover. Choose one that's acetone-free so it won't leave the nails dried out.
2 Use an emery board to file the nails into a smooth oval shape. If they're long, use a nail clipper first – it's faster and puts less strain on the delicate nailbed. File towards the centre, as filing down the side or back and forth weakens the nails and encourages splitting.
3 Massage cuticle softener (almond oil is a good alternative) into the base of each nail for ten to twenty seconds. Then, using an orange stick wrapped in cotton wool, gently push back each cuticle and ease away any dirt or dead skin.
4 Take a little exfoliator – if you don't want to splash out on one specifically for the hands, a face or body scrub will do – and use each thumb to buff from wrist to fingertips. Remember to include the nails, backs of the hands and between your fingers.
5 Rinse your hands clean in a bowl of warm water and pat them dry with a towel.
6 Finish by applying a nourishing hand cream or lotion to replenish and soften the skin – try our quick *Handy Work* massage (on page 178) for added indulgence. If your hands feel slippery afterwards, blot the excess moisturizer with a tissue.

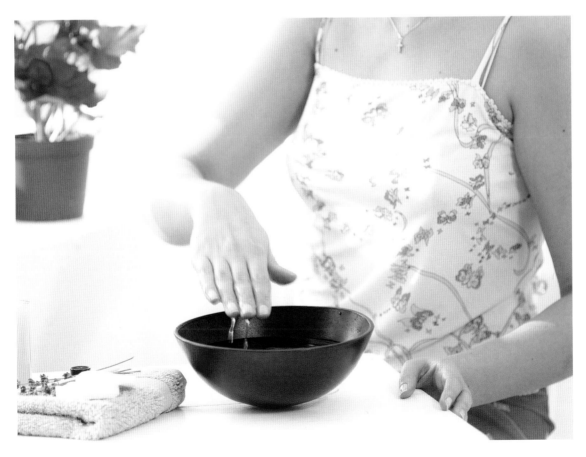

Handy Work

A simple hand massage is one of the most effective ways to de-stress. Taking each hand in turn, use the opposite thumb to apply pressure in small circles clockwise around the palm. Finish on the small mound of muscle just below where your thumb and forefinger meet, spending an extra minute on this acupressure point which is used to release tension and focus the mind. Repeat the movements on the back of your hand, then use the thumb and forefinger to gently massage each finger from base to tip.

Three Top Hand-care Tips

- Wear rubber gloves for cleaning and gardening – they may not look glamorous, but neither does weathered skin and peeling nails.
- Keep hand lotion where you can see it – by the sink, next to your alarm clock, or on your desk. You'll remember to apply it and you can take a few seconds out to relax if you massage the lotion in.
- Choose a hand cream that incorporates skincare technology: those boasting sunscreens and anti-ageing ingredients can protect against fine lines and brown spots as well as help treat any signs already there.

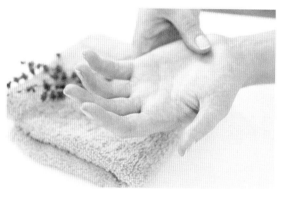

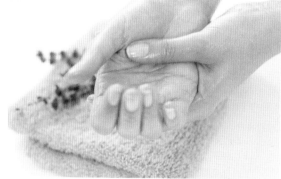

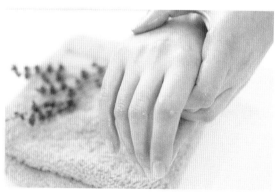

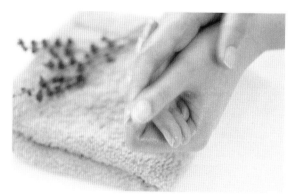

Fighting Nail Imperfections

The nails on both hands and feet can easily fall foul of a number of problems. Below are a few of the most common and how to treat them.

Yellowing

Any nail polish (be it a pale or dark shade) can leave behind a yellow tinge if applied directly to the nails. To prevent this, always use one or two layers of base coat first when colouring the nails; if the stain is already there, use a three-way buffer every few days until it has disappeared.

White Spots

In most cases, a simple knock can be injury enough to prevent the soft cells that form the nails from bonding together properly, leaving a white mark instead of transparency. These spots cannot be removed so leave them to grow out naturally.

Grooves and Ridges

Again, injury is the most common cause of irregularity in the smoothness of the nails and must be left to grow out. As this takes several months, you can minimize their appearance by gently buffing the nails when they are clean and applying a ridge-filler before you use nail polish.

Splitting or Flaking

Dehydration is the main culprit when nails start to split or flake. Water swells the 'glue' that bonds together the cells of the nail, weakening it even when dry again. Protect your nails from getting wet by using rubber gloves wherever possible and applying a hand cream or sweet almond oil to replenish moisture levels.

If you are concerned that any irregularities in your nails may be due to more serious medical conditions such as psoriasis or a fungal infection, book an appointment with an accredited dermatologist. If the problem is related to your feet, see a registered chiropodist or podiatrist.

Exercises for the Feet

The feet are the foundation on which we stand, and like the foundations of a house they play a very important role. You would not dream of building a house on unsound foundations and the feet deserve the same respect.

The average adult has a walking stride of approximately one metre during which the foot impacts, bends, stretches and twists under our weight. This occurs about 1,000 times for each mile, and most of us clock up about 700 miles of walking a year. That's a lot of footwork in a lifetime.

The foot is a very intricate structure composed of many small bones, muscles, ligaments and tendons. It supports the weight of the body and must be flexible enough to cope with all surfaces, walking on pebbles, rocks or sand, for example, but rigid enough to provide a lever for pushing off when running, for example. The feet are in essence shock absorbers.

They also play an important role in our vascular system. There are various blood 'pumps' in the lower leg. The foot pump is different from the calf pump because it is not affected by ankle or toe movement. Those in the foot are on the plantar lateral, the underneath outside part of the foot, which means they get flattened under our body weight every time we walk. This flattening, which is followed by expansion as the body weight is released, produces the 'pump' effect of these veins and a column of blood can thus be directed up to the heart. So walking really is good for your circulation.

It's a good idea to restrict your wearing of high heels to only the most necessary occasions as they play havoc with your posture. Trainers are great footwear, but do remember to walk barefoot sometimes. The soles of the feet are a vital part of our sensory biofeedback system. They need stimulating, and when we walk barefoot they send messages throughout the body affecting our overall balance and posture. Medical research is just realizing the importance of this sensory feedback with regard to back problems.

When standing, you need to think of a triangle or tripod at the base of each foot. Mentally draw a triangle on each foot from the base of the big toe to the base of the small toe to the centre of the heel. You need to ground yourself on those two triangles with the weight centred evenly on them.

These foot exercises will wake up your feet and ensure that the spring stays in your step.

The Mexican Wave

Aim
To work the toes individually.

Starting Position
As above.

Action
It's quite simple really. One by one lift the toes, starting with the big toe, and Mexican wave down to the little toe, then reverse the wave.

Watchpoints for Isolating the Toes and Mexican Wave
- Keep the bones at the base of your toes (the metatarsals) flat on the floor.
- Don't let the heel come off the floor.
- Don't let the feet roll.

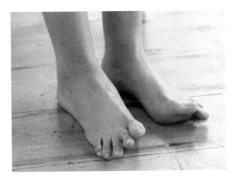

Towel Dragging

Equipment
A towel.

Aim
To work the arches, helping to prevent flat feet.

Starting Position
Put the towel on the floor in front of you and then sit tall on a sturdy chair. Place one foot on the towel, keep the leg in good alignment: in a line with your knees and hips (you don't want to be twisting at all).

Action
1. Keeping the toes long and not letting them scrunch up, drag the towel towards you. As you lift the toes, spread them wide, but leave the metatarsal bones down. Grab the towel with the ball of your foot, pulling it towards you. Spread the toes and release, then drag again.
2. Repeat eight times with each foot.
3. To make it harder you can place a weight on the towel.

Watchpoints
- Do not allow the feet to roll in or out.
- It's very tempting just to screw the toes up but that's not the idea, make those arches work.
- If your foot cramps rest and try again later.

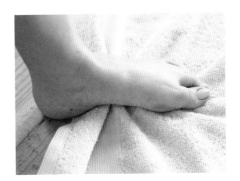

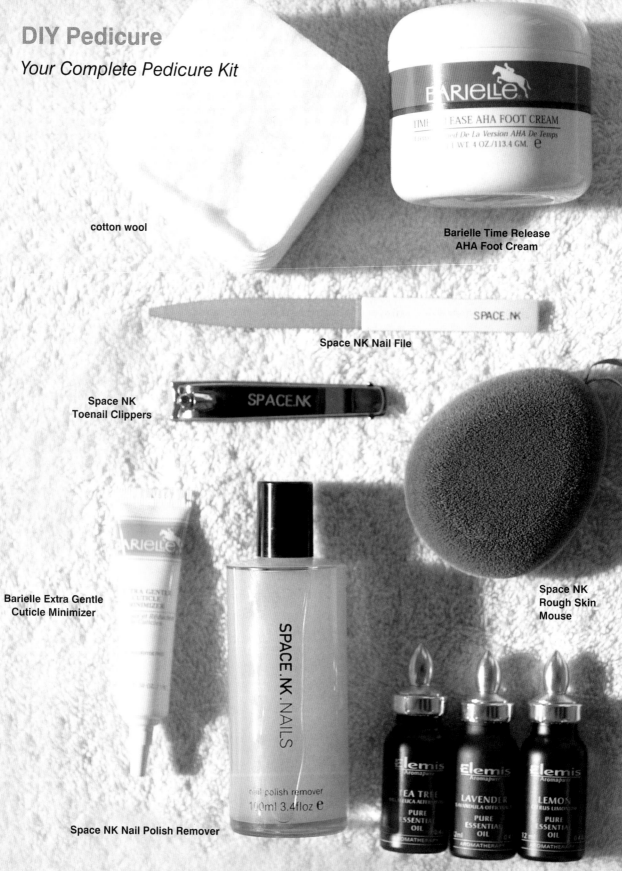

DIY Pedicure

Your Complete Pedicure Kit

cotton wool

Barielle Time Release
AHA Foot Cream

Space NK Nail File

Space NK
Toenail Clippers

Barielle Extra Gentle
Cuticle Minimizer

Space NK
Rough Skin
Mouse

Space NK Nail Polish Remover

Elemis Pure Essential Oils in Lemon, Tea Tree and Lavender

Pedicure Masterclass

Our feet take an amazing 18,000 steps every day so it's ironic that they receive such little attention. Redress the balance by treating your feet to this revitalizing monthly pedicure.

1 Get rid of any old nail varnish with an acetone-free polish remover and cotton wool.

2 Add a few drops of essential oil (try deodorizing tea tree, uplifting peppermint or healing lavender) to a basin of warm water and soak the feet for five minutes.

3 While they are soaking, take each one in turn and use an exfoliator to remove any dead, hard skin, paying special attention to heels and soles. Choose from one of the great foot scrubs, files or pumice stones available for super smoothness.

4 Dry the feet thoroughly (especially between the toes to prevent athlete's foot), then use a pair of nail clippers to trim the toenails straight across. Cutting them too short can cause toenails to ingrow, so smooth down rough edges and corners with an emery board.

5 Massage a cuticle softener into the base of each nail for ten to twenty seconds, then use an orange stick wrapped in cotton wool to push back each cuticle and gently clean the base of the nail, down each side and under the tip.

6 Apply a pea-sized amount of nourishing foot cream and spend a few minutes massaging it in. For a really relaxing finish, ask a friend or partner to treat you to our Reflexology Basics technique (on page 184).

Reflexology Basics

As well as bringing respite to weary, worn-out feet, a massage can benefit the entire body. According to reflexology, the foot is like a map with each area, filled with nerve endings, corresponding to a particular part of the body. Foot reflexology is the skill of applying gentle pressure to the reflexes on the soles of the feet, restoring the body's natural flow of energy to stimulate self-healing while promoting relaxation and wellbeing.

This massage sequence has been created by Louise Keet. A top reflexologist from the renowned Keet Clinic in London, Louise is also a principal of the Central London School of Reflexology. The sequence has been designed to help easily identify the points on the feet that relate to stress management. To reap the full benefits, ask a friend or partner to treat you to this simple technique, then return the favour, however, if you are pregnant or under the care of a medical practitioner, seek a qualified reflexologist.

Take off your shoes and socks, then lie comfortably on a bed. Your partner should sit at the end of the bed and apply a small amount of powder to your feet. Using the chart, ask them to follow these steps, applying gentle pressure.

1   Begin with this relaxation technique to put your partner at ease. The first contact you have is important so, starting with the right leg, use both hands to massage up the leg and down through the toes. Repeat on the left leg.
2   Taking the right foot, support the big toe with the fingers of your left hand and use your right thumb to caterpillar walk up from the base of the toe to the top. Walk up in lines so that you cover the entire surface. The base of the big toe corresponds to the neck – the rest of the toe to the head. At the centre, you will pass the pituitary gland that helps regulate hormones, including your metabolism and response to stress. Repeat on the left foot, using the right hand for support and applying pressure with the left thumb.
3   Support the right foot with one hand and walk across the diaphragm line with the thumb of the other hand. Often, you will take shallower breaths when stressed and this affects the diaphragm – a relaxed person takes deep breaths. Repeat on the left foot.
4   The stomach can suffer greatly as a result of stress. Work lightly over the stomach reflex to rebalance it. Use your left hand to support the right foot. Caterpillar walk with your right thumb, starting just below the diaphragm line and moving up to its centre. Repeat for three lines. Repeat on the left foot, using the right hand for support and making the movements with your left thumb.
5   As stress can affect the body's immune system, the lymphatic system is important for building up resistance to disease. Use your index finger and thumb, placing them at the base of the second and third toe of the right foot. Walk three steps towards the ankle, hold the pressure and slide back out through the toes. Repeat in between all of the toes, then do the same on the left foot.
6   Place the right thumb on the solar plexus point of the left foot and the left thumb on the solar plexus point of the right foot. Ask your partner to breathe in, push into the points and breathe out. Repeat for three breaths.
7   Finish by wrapping the feet in a towel and let your partner relax for ten minutes. Offer them a glass of water to help flush any toxins out of the body.

For details of the Keet Clinic and the Central London School of Reflexology, see the Directory on page 214.

Stress Management

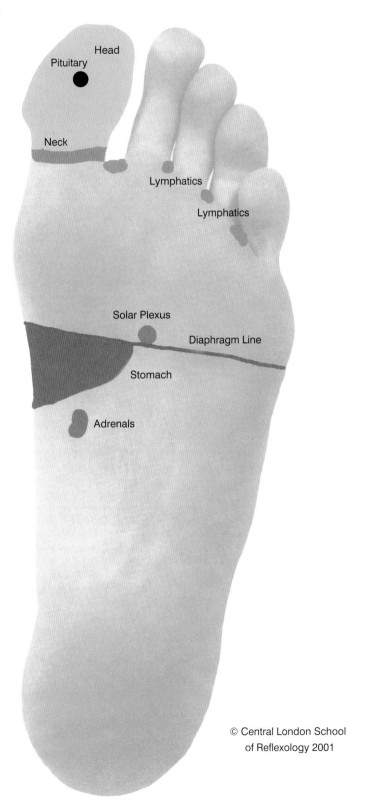

Head
Pituitary
Neck
Lymphatics
Lymphatics
Solar Plexus
Diaphragm Line
Stomach
Adrenals

© Central London School
of Reflexology 2001

Create Your Own Floral Foot Soak

In Bali, the foot soak is traditionally used to help restore balance and, if it has flowers added, it washes away bad luck. It's also a beautiful start to many of their spa treatments. To calm the senses and relieve aching feet, try this simple Indonesian technique: fill a large bowl with warm water and add freshly picked, aromatic flowers such as rose, lavender and geranium, along with a few drops of cooling lemongrass essential oil. Sit back, unwind and soak your feet for ten to fifteen minutes.

Top Five Foot Treats

Molton Brown Thermalsalt Foot Soak

Body Shop Lemongrass
Deodorising Foot Polish

Origins Sole Searcher Smoothing
Foot Scrub

Decleor Beauté des Pieds
Foot Care Cream

Aveda Foot Relief

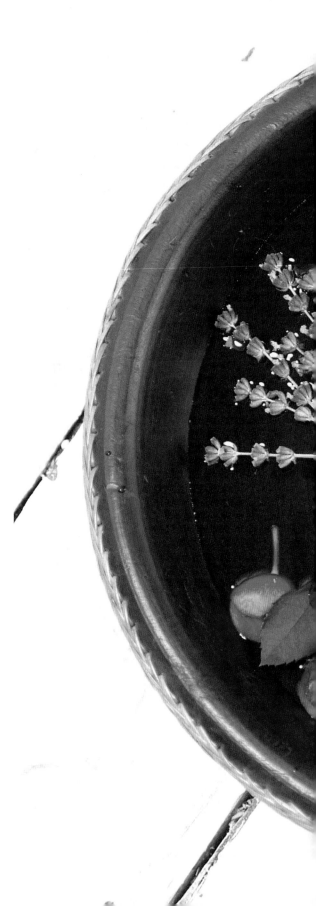

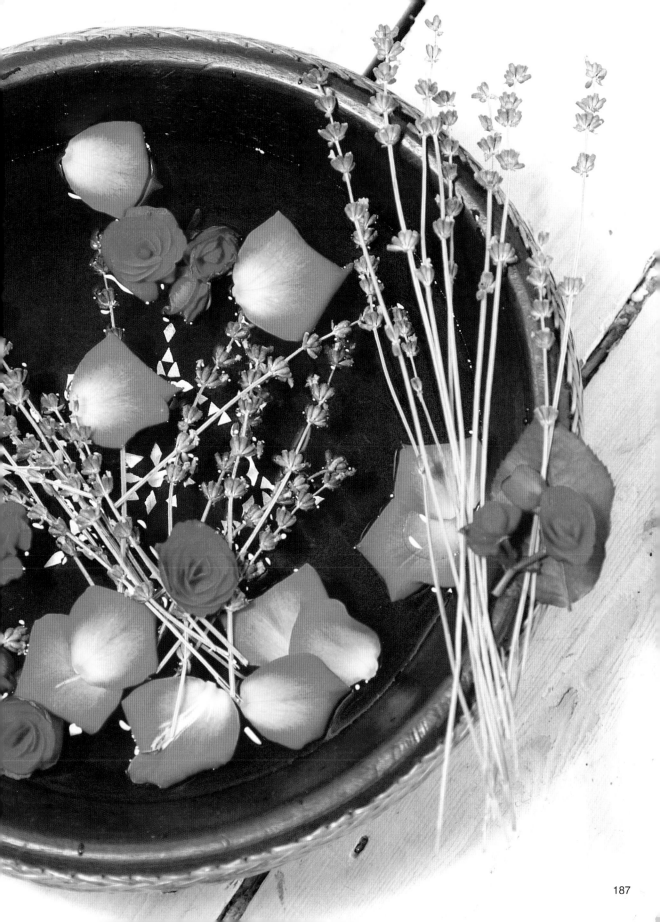

WINDING DOWN
at the end of each
day should precede
flopping straight into bed.
The body needs time to
unwind and slow down after
working, exercising and
socializing so that it can fully
benefit from a good night's
sleep and ensure that
you are refreshed and
rejuvenated the following
morning. Making this time
a ritual of relaxation and
reflection will help you
reap mental, physical and
spiritual rewards.

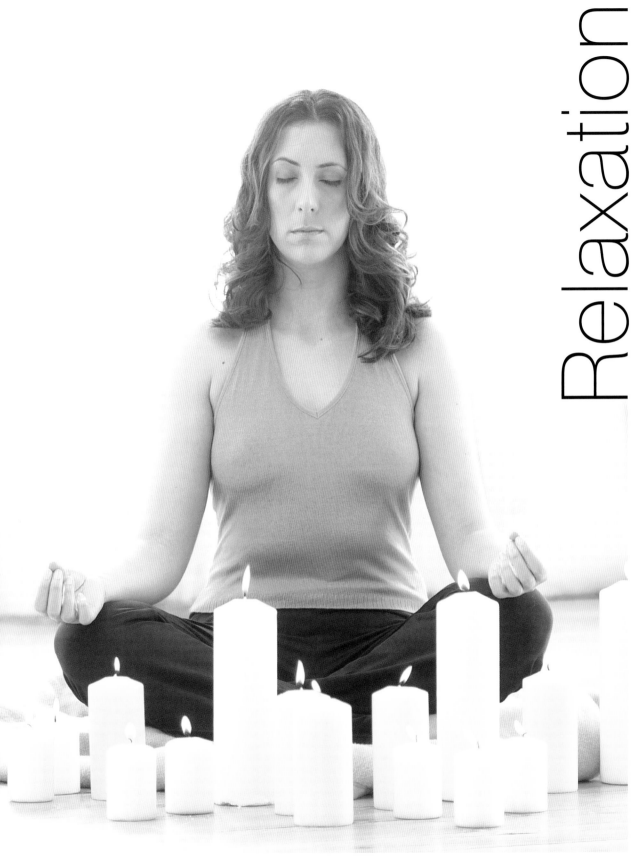

Relaxation

Exercises for Relaxation

The following exercises have been chosen for their ability to ease tension out of tight, tired muscles, to rebalance the muscles after the day's activities and also to focus and still the mind.

Studio Stretch

This exercise is very good for stilling the mind.

Aim
To stretch the inner thighs and the spine gently.

Equipment
Large cushion (optional)

Starting Position
Sit with your knees bent and the soles of your feet together. Do not bring the feet too close to you, you should be comfortable. Your pelvis should be square. You could sit with your back to a wall to check this. If you wish you may try sitting on the edge of a large cushion, it will help the alignment of your spine.

Action
1 Breathe in to prepare and lengthen up through the spine.
2 Breathe out, zip up and hollow, lift up out of your hips and move up and over an imaginary beach ball.
3 Take twelve breaths, breathing into your lower ribcage and back.
4 Relax into the stretch edging forward if you can, still hollowing.
5 Your arms are resting in front of you, your neck is long, your shoulder blades are resting down into your back.
6 After twelve breaths, slowly uncurl on the out-breath, zipping up and hollowing, and rebuilding the spine vertebra by vertebra.

Watchpoints
• Try to think of all the bony bumps of the spine (like a dinosaur's back) opening and separating.

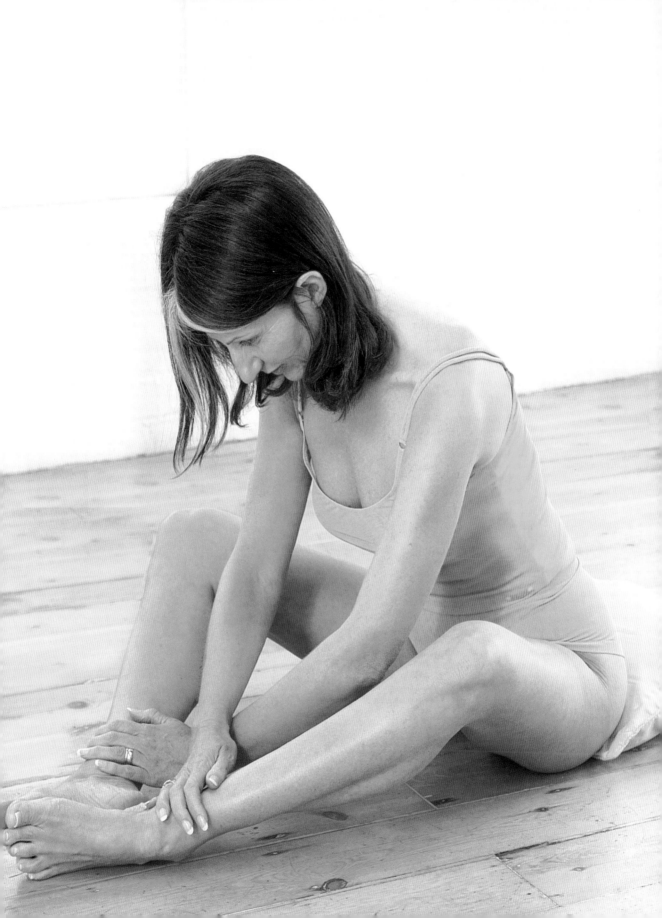

Circle of Chalk (*intermediate*)

Aim

To open the upper body and sides, stretching out the pectoral muscles. To rotate the spine safely with stability, working from a strong centre.

This exercise has the most wonderful feel-good factor. Perfect at the end of a bad day, or even a good day.

Equipment

A large pillow.
A small cushion (optional).

Starting Position

Lie on your side with a pillow under your head – a bed pillow is perfect. Have your back in a straight line but curl your knees up to hip level. Extend your arms in front of you, in line with your shoulders, palms together. You may like to place a small cushion between your knees – it helps keep good pelvic alignment.

> **Warning:** if you have a neck, shoulder or a disc injury, please consult your practitioner before starting this exercise.

Action

1 Breathe in to prepare and lengthen through the spine.
2 Breathe out and zip up and hollow. Imagining you have a piece of chalk in your hand, reach the top arm beyond the lower arm, taking your hand above you and round your head. Allow your head to move naturally, following the opening movement of the shoulders. The knees stay together and the centre is strong.
3 Breathing normally, reach your hand right round as if you are drawing a circle on the floor. It will pass behind you, down over your buttocks and back up to join the other hand.
4 Repeat five times on each side. The aim is to keep the hand in contact with the floor but, as that's difficult, please work within your comfort range.

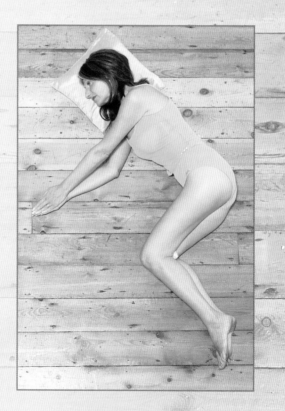

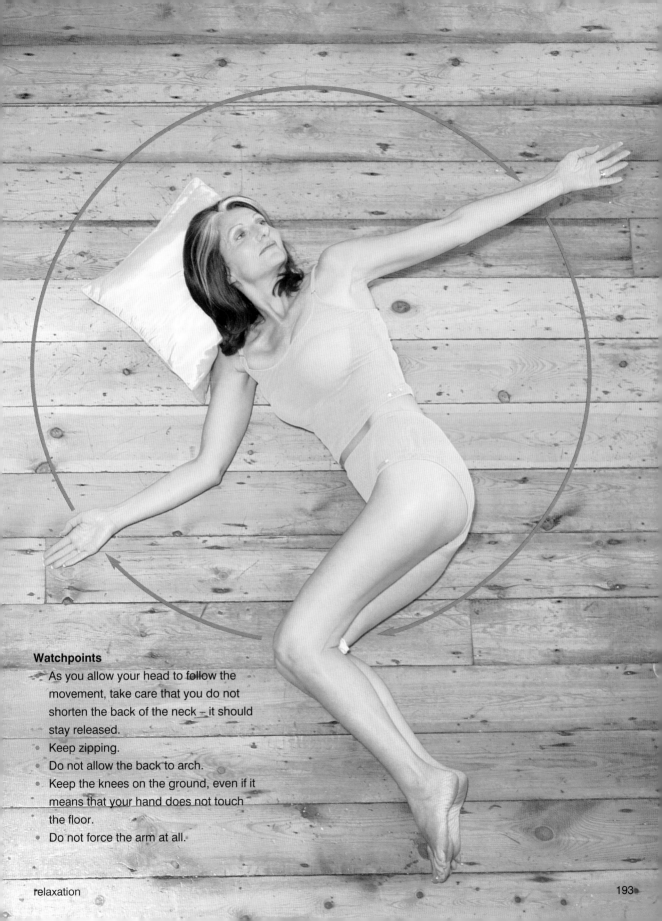

Watchpoints

- As you allow your head to follow the movement, take care that you do not shorten the back of the neck – it should stay released.
- Keep zipping.
- Do not allow the back to arch.
- Keep the knees on the ground, even if it means that your hand does not touch the floor.
- Do not force the arm at all.

Shoulder Drops

A wonderful exercise that allows you to let go of any tension around the shoulders and neck. Great to do at the end of a stress-filled day.

Aim

To release tension in the upper body.

Starting Position

Lie in the Relaxation Position (see page 14).
Gently roll your head from side to side as described for Neck Rolls on page 28.

Action

1 Raise both arms towards the ceiling directly above your shoulders, palms facing.
2 Reach for the ceiling with one arm, stretch through the fingertips. The shoulder blade comes off the floor. Then drop the arm back down into the floor.
3 Repeat ten times with each arm. Feel your upper back widening and the tension in your shoulders releasing down into the floor.

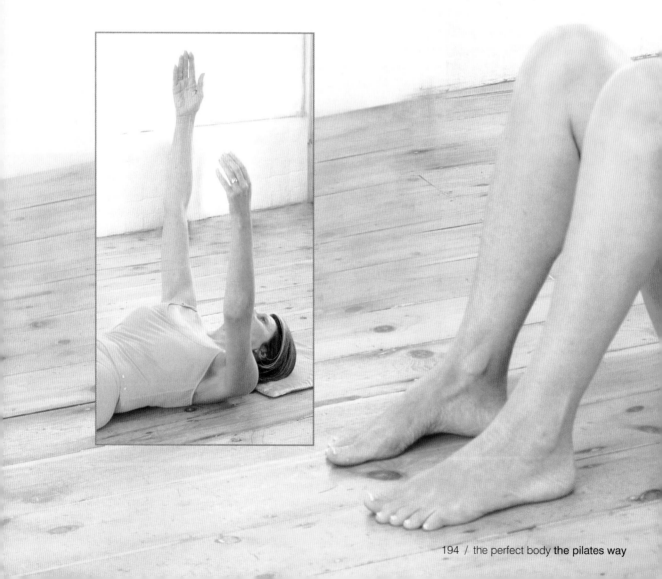

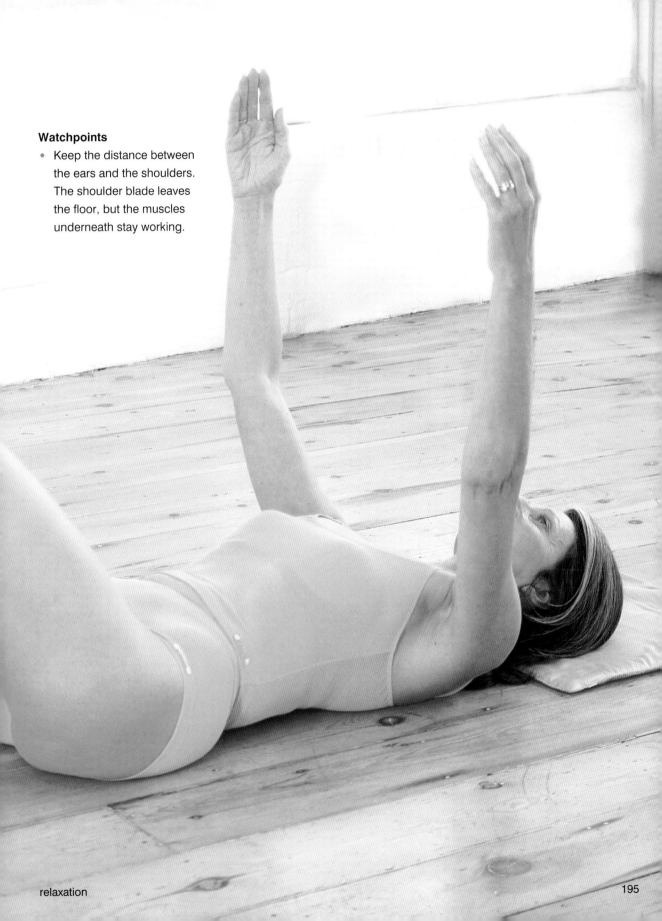

Watchpoints

- Keep the distance between the ears and the shoulders. The shoulder blade leaves the floor, but the muscles underneath stay working.

Hip Flexor Stretch

Aim

To lengthen the hip flexors gently. If you sit all day, it is likely that your hip flexor muscles will shorten, which affects the angle of your pelvis by pulling anteriorly.

Starting Position

Lie in the Relaxation Position (see page 14).

Action

1 Breathe in wide and full to prepare.
2 Breathe out, zip up and hollow. Keeping that sense of hollowness in the pelvis, hinge the right knee up to your chest, dropping the thigh bone down into the hip joint.
3 Breathe in, as you clasp the right leg below the knee or under the thigh. If you have any knee problems clasp the leg under the thigh rather than below the knee so that the joint is not compressed.

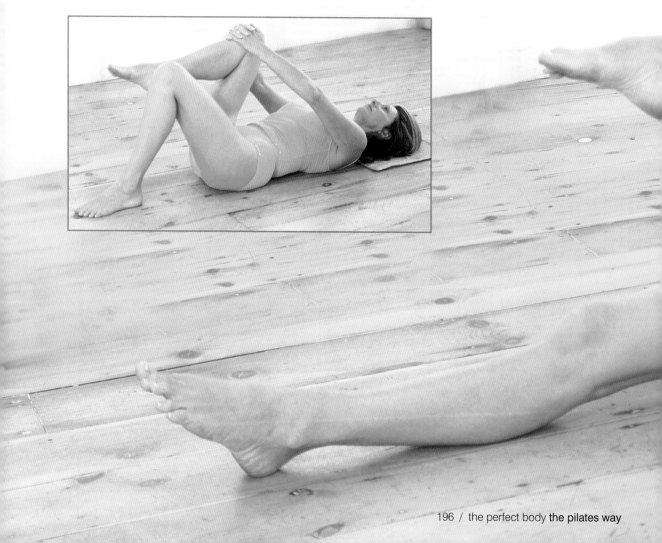

4 Breathe out, still zipping, and stretch the left leg along the floor. Your lower back should remain in neutral. If it arches, bend the left knee back up again a little. Hold this stretch for five breaths.

5 Breathe in as you slide the leg back.

6 Breathe out and zip up and hollow, as you lower the right bent knee to the floor, keeping the abdominals engaged.

7 Repeat twice on each side, keeping your shoulders relaxed and down.

Watchpoints

• Check the position of the upper body, elbows open, breastbone soft, shoulder blades down into the back, neck released.

• Are you in neutral?

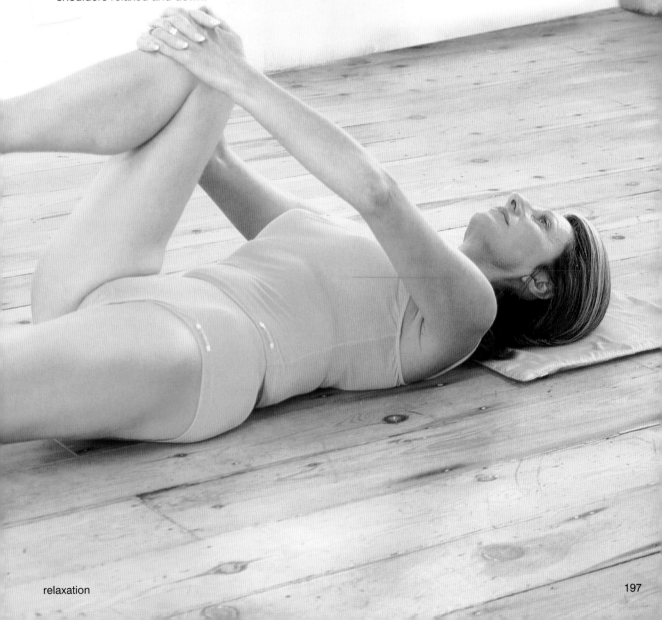

A Short Relaxation

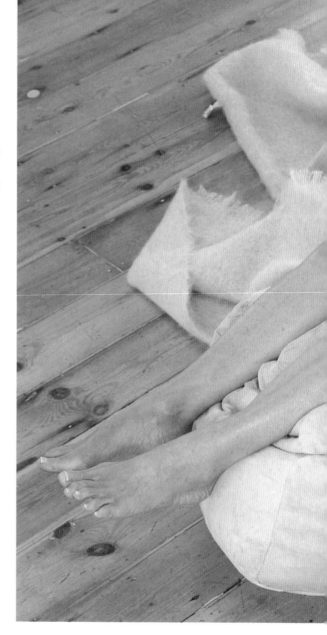

Aim

Use this technique to recognize and release tension from the body – it's the perfect way to end the day or any of your workout sessions. Ideally, you should persuade a friend to read the instructions aloud to you, otherwise try taping them.

Equipment

A large pillow (optional).

Starting Position

Lie in the Relaxation Position (see page 14), and allow your whole body to melt down into the floor, lengthening and widening. Place a large pillow under your knees, if you want.

Action

1 Take your awareness down to your feet and soften the soles, uncurling the toes.
2 Soften your ankles.
3 Soften your calves.
4 Release your knees.
5 Release your thighs.
6 Allow your hips to open.
7 Allow the small of your back to sink into the floor as though you are sinking down into the folds of a hammock.
8 Feel the length of your spine.
9 Take your awareness down to your hands, stretch your fingers away from your palms, feel the centre of your palms opening.
10 Allow the fingers to curl, the palms to soften.
11 Allow your elbows to open.
12 Allow the front of your shoulders to soften.
13 With each out breath allow your shoulder blades to widen.
14 Allow your breastbone to soften.
15 Allow your neck to release.
16 Check your jaw: it should be loose and free.
17 Allow your tongue to widen at its base and rest comfortably at the bottom of your mouth.
18 Your lips are softly closed.
19 Your eyes are softly closed.
20 Your forehead is wide and smooth and completely free of lines.
21 Your face feels soft.
22 Your body feels soft and warm.
23 Your spine is gently released down into the floor.
24 Observe your breathing, but do not interrupt it. Simply enjoy its natural rhythm.

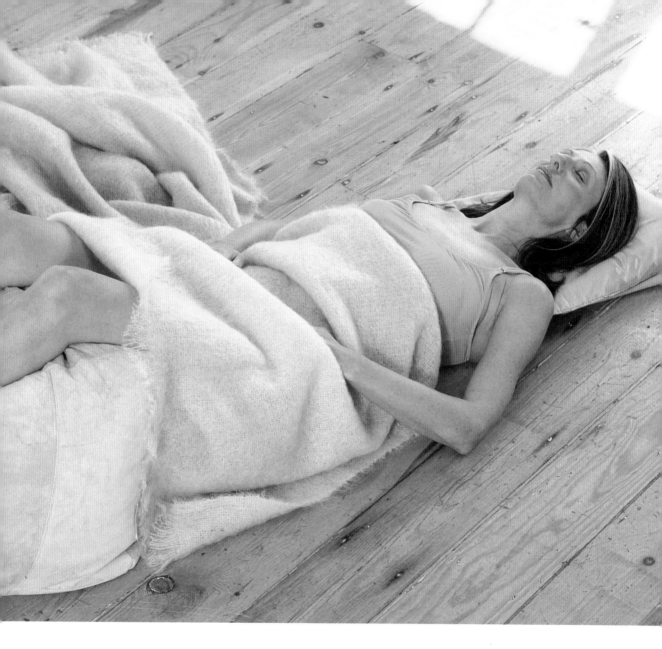

To Come Out of the Relaxation

* Very gently allow your head to roll to one side, allowing its own weight to move it.
* Slowly come back to the centre and allow it to roll to the other side, then bring it back to the centre again.
* Wriggle your fingers and then your toes.
* Very slowly roll on to one side and rest there for a few minutes before slowly getting up.

Chill-out Techniques

Sometimes it takes more than a hot drink and five minutes with your feet up to feel completely relaxed. To ease mind and muscle tension before you go to bed, try alternating or combining these three wonderful ways of unwinding.

Aromatherapy Massage

Aromatherapy massage is a relaxation triple whammy. Firstly, the massage movements ease tight muscles and release tension from top to toe. Secondly, as the aromatherapy oils are applied to the skin, you inhale their scent – tiny molecules that affect your mood and sense of wellbeing. Thirdly, the oils are absorbed through the skin into the body, promoting physical benefits.

Choosing the right blend of essential oils is crucial. Eschew stimulating oils such as rosemary, bergamot and peppermint in favour of those that are calming and comforting. Camomile, lavender, neroli, ylang ylang and rose are all great choices (with aromatherapy you get what you pay for, so buy high quality). Try one of the fantastic blends from renowned companies such as Aveda, ESPA, Elemis and Origins, or mix twenty drops of essential oil with 10mls of a carrier oil such as evening primrose, almond or coconut.

As it takes a minimum of twenty minutes for the oils to be absorbed, the ideal time span for an aromatherapy massage is about one hour. If you are doing it yourself, aim for at least twenty minutes. The easiest way to perform self-massage is by standing up (with a chair beside you for support) and following this easy routine:

1 Warm a little of the oil between your palms and cup them over your face. Inhale and exhale slowly three times, breathing in the aroma. Try to relax all the muscles up and down your body while you do this.

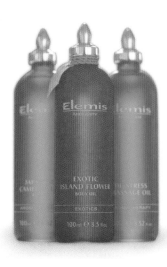

2 Place your fingertips along your hairline and gently massage towards the crown, then move down to the back of the neck with firm, circular movements. Use your forefinger to massage behind the ears, then gently rub both ears and earlobes between your forefinger and thumb.

3 Starting at the chin, use the circular movements along the jawline, across the cheeks and nose, then up and over the forehead. Massage around the eyes with your middle finger. Begin at the inner corner and follow the orbit, pressing gently underneath, then above each eye. Repeat three times.

4 Move down to your feet and start using an easy massage technique called effleurage – long strokes up and down with the palms of the hands. Massage each leg in turn, then the bottom, stomach, chest, arms and shoulders. Add a little more oil each time you move to a different part of the body.

5 If you can reach (or have a willing partner), include the back too. You can also add the massage techniques in Back Rub Bliss (see page 90). When you have finished, sit down and take a few minutes to relax.

> **Warning:** most essential oils and massage techniques are not suitable for use during pregnancy. For further advice, consult your doctor or an accredited aromatherapist.

Deep Breathing

Oxygen is fundamental to our whole being, yet most of us have forgotten how to breathe properly. Bad posture, pollution and a frenetic lifestyle combine to rob us of oxygen's vital energy, but correct breathing can instantly revitalize the body as well as calming the senses. Different methods of breathing are suited to different activities – for example we use lateral breathing during Pilates, but deep breathing which expands the lungs and stomach is most beneficial for relaxation.

- Eliminate distractions and interruptions such as the phone, radio, television and other people. Make sure the room is warm, softly lit (candles are ideal) and cosy.
- Sit comfortably on a chair with both feet flat on the floor, or cross-legged on a pillow. Keep your back straight, your eyes closed and relax the jaw and facial muscles.
- Breathe in through your nose, expanding your stomach rather than your chest as you inhale. (You might find this easier if you place one hand on your stomach and watch it rise and fall.) Think of your lungs filling with air in every direction a bit like a balloon filling up.
- Gently and slowly, allow the breath to flow out through the mouth. Exhale for twice as long as you inhale, breathing out until you have completely emptied the lungs of stale air.
- Concentrate on the smooth, rhythmic sound of your breath for five minutes before slowly opening your eyes and becoming aware of your surroundings.

Meditation

Once you have reacquainted your body with the tranquillizing effects of deep breathing, take it a step further with this simple method of meditating. Practised regularly, it can reduce blood pressure, heart rate and stress levels, leaving the mind clearer, the body rejuvenated and energies more focused. Aim to meditate for fifteen to twenty minutes: if you find it difficult to concentrate without distraction at first, build up the time over a week.

- Sit as you would for deep breathing, in a tranquil place and in a comfortable position.
- One by one, empty your mind of the worries accumulated during the day until you can focus on a single positive thought, image or affirmation.
- If you prefer, repeat the traditional Sanskrit mantra 'om' (drawn out into a long sound) either aloud or in your head.
- When you wish to finish, gradually become aware of your surroundings – first the sounds, the smells and then the sights around you. Stand up slowly, then start to move around at your own pace.

With proper instruction, deep meditation can benefit every part of your life. If you want to explore its power, join a local class for Raja yoga or trans-cendental meditation, or go on a retreat to fully immerse yourself.

Sweet Slumber

Beauty sleep is not an old wives' tale: your body needs a nightly average of eight hours to repair, regenerate and revitalize. Partying hard – with the additional damage done by smoking, drinking and not eating properly – leaves the body struggling to feed its organs (including the skin) with blood, while the hormones that keep us feeling happy, convert food into energy and promote growth, fail to replenish.

Dreaming – which only happens during deep or rapid eye movement sleep – is also thought to be good for the mind, helping release tension and anxiety. The result of long-term sleep deprivation is poor concentration, a lacklustre complexion, increased levels of stress and diminished tissue repair and muscle function.

The time you go to bed is critical too. Recent research has shown that the body works harder to achieve its critical sleep goals between 10 p.m. and midnight – so staying up and sleeping late isn't a substitute. The relaxation techniques on the previous pages combined with the ideas here should help you prepare for a rejuvenating night's sleep.

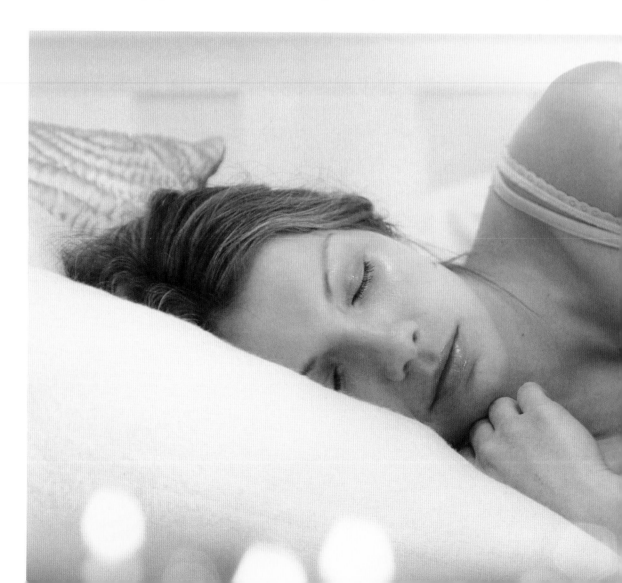

- Make your bed comfortable and inviting. Surround yourself with fluffy duvets, blankets, sheets, cushions and pillows in soft colours and soothing textures such as silk, brushed cotton and fleece.
- Ensure your pillow is the right height. Your head and shoulders should be at right angles to each other so you don't strain the muscles in your neck.
- Keep the room well ventilated but with a moderate temperature. If the room is too hot, you'll be restless; too cold and you won't be able to relax.
- Additionally, if the room is too light, wear eyeshades; if it's too noisy, use soft earplugs.

Scents for Serenity

Maximize your relaxation time by creating an atmosphere of calm in your bedroom, bathroom or living room. Light a favourite aromatherapy candle or vaporize ten drops of a good-quality essential oil, mixed with water. Try one of these uplifting oils to help you unwind:

- lavender
- neroli
- geranium
- rose
- ylang ylang

Eating for Good Sleep

What you eat has a direct effect on your quality of sleep. Comfort foods – usually carbohydrates such as pasta, bread and potatoes – tell the brain to release serotonin, a mood-enhancing hormone that encourages the body to slow down and relax, whereas fatty foods take many hours to digest. Certain foods have hidden stimulants – red meats and vegetables such as aubergine and spinach contain amino acids that can keep you awake. If you find it hard to avoid such foods, especially when eating out, enjoy your meal but only eat limited amounts of these ingredients. Try applying these successful slumber tips too:

- A carbohydrate-rich meal is relaxing; a protein-rich meal is stimulating. Eat a larger portion of carbohydrates than protein at dinner.
- Have a light meal in the evening and eat at least three hours before you go to bed so your food can digest.
- Going to bed hungry will keep you awake too, so a bedtime snack can assist sleep. Two hours before, try a carbohydrate-rich snack such as cereal or wholemeal toast.

Foods to Stock Up On

- Wholemeal bread and pasta, brown rice, couscous and potatoes: rich in carbohydrates that encourage the production of serotonin, soothing the body and helping to regulate sleep.
- Bananas, figs and dates: rich in the amino acid tryptophan, used to make serotonin.
- Avocados: rich in vitamin B6, essential for the production of tryptophan.
- Warm milk: soothing and relaxing. Milk is also rich in calcium and magnesium, which help to relax the muscles.
- Peppermint tea: aids smooth digestion.

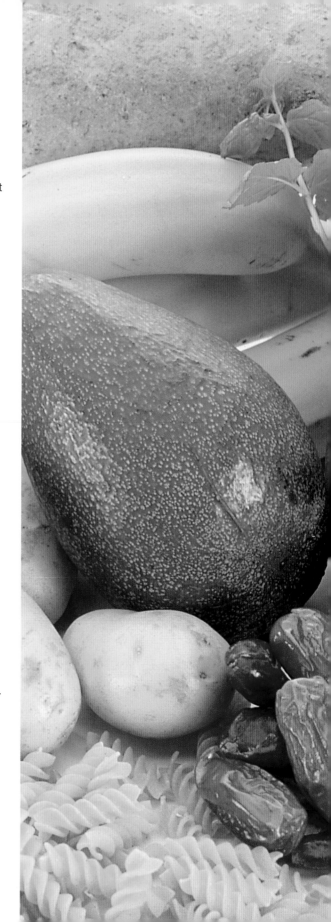

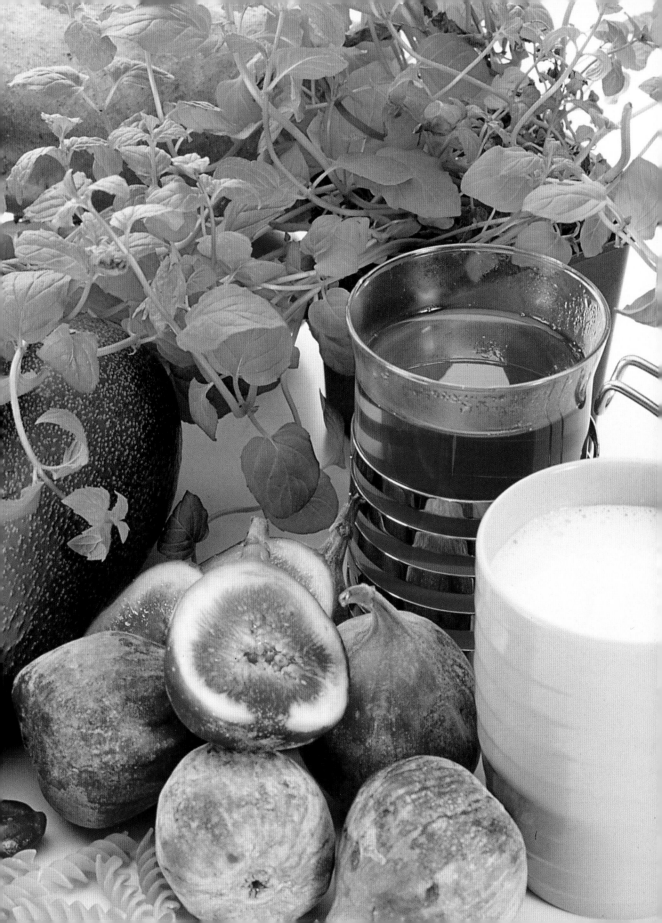

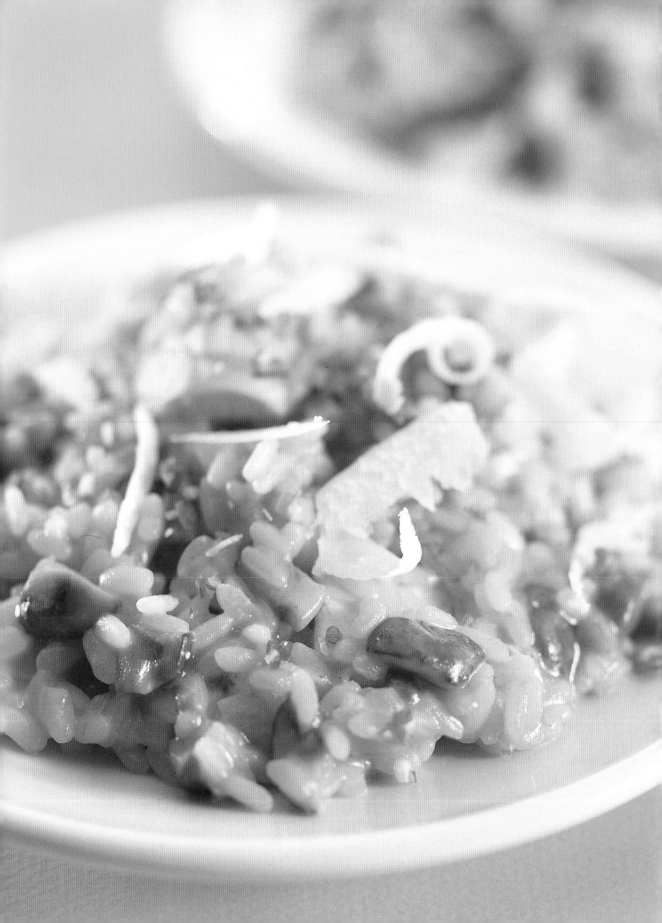

Chicken and Mushroom Risotto

Preparation time: **15 minutes**
Cooking time: **30 minutes**
Serves: **4**

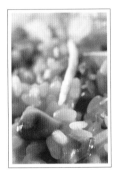

2 cooked chicken breasts

2 tbsp olive oil

1 onion, finely chopped

250g brown cap mushrooms, roughly chopped

225g arborio (risotto) rice

salt and ground black pepper

1 litre hot chicken or vegetable stock

50g Parmesan cheese, freshly grated

juice and zest of ½ lemon

shavings of fresh Parmesan

spring onion, finely chopped

Remove the skin from the chicken and discard. Chop the flesh into bite-sized pieces.

Heat the oil in a large saucepan, add the onion and fry over medium heat for about 3 minutes or until it begins to soften. Add the mushrooms and continue to cook for a further 3 minutes. Add the rice and seasoning stirring continually for 1–2 minutes.

Add just enough stock to cover the rice and stir frequently until most of the stock has been absorbed. Continue adding the stock in this way until it is almost completely absorbed and the rice is tender.

Stir in the chicken and cook for a further 1–2 minutes or until hot. Remove from the heat and stir in the grated Parmesan, lemon juice and zest.

Garnish with the shavings of fresh Parmesan and the spring onions and serve immediately.

Vegetarian option: omit the chicken and increase the quantity of mushrooms to 350g. A few dried mushrooms, reconstituted in a little warm water, will give the risotto a deliciously intense mushroom flavour. Follow the instructions on the packet.

Hot Carob Drink

Preparation time: **5 minutes**
Cooking time: **5 minutes**
Serves: **2**

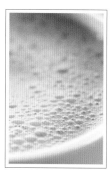

300ml semi-skimmed milk
25g unsweetened carob or plain chocolate bar, grated
5ml (1 tsp) clear honey
pinch of ground cinnamon

Pour the milk into a small saucepan and heat gently.
Whisk in the remaining ingredients. Pour into mugs
and serve immediately.

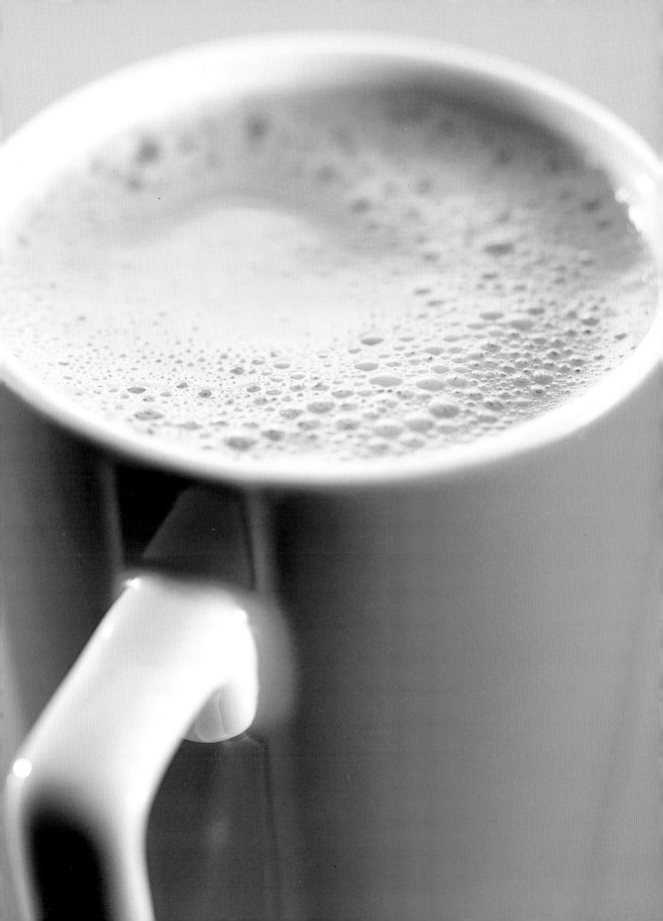

The following Pilates workouts are approximately 40 minutes in length and are perfectly balanced. Try to do five different workouts each week. Where an exercise has different levels, work at whichever level is suitable for you.

Remember to do at least three 20–30 minute sessions of cardiovascular training each week as well. Aerobic activity improves your body's ability to transport oxygen. We have already seen how the body's fat tissues have a very low metabolic rate: they do not burn calories, only muscle cells do this. Therefore, the more muscle tissues you have, the better you will burn calories. However, you need oxygen to do this – the more oxygen your muscles receive via the bloodstream the more calories and fat you will burn.

Here are some suggestions for aerobic activity:

- brisk/power walking

- jogging
  (treadmill / outdoor)

- swimming

- cycling
  (stationary / outdoor)

- rollerblading

- trampolining

- spinning
  (instructor-led class)

- kick boxing

- dancing

- skiing

- aerobics class

- cross training (machine)

- rowing (indoor/outdoor)

And whenever possible, walk rather than drive, use the stairs rather than the lift, consider going upstairs on the bus.

Workouts

Workouts

Aveda (*www.aveda.com*)
Hip, eco-conscious beauty and lifestyle line, focusing on natural skincare, haircare, make-up and fragrance.

Barielle (*www.barielle.com*)
The experts in professional-quality treatment products for hands, nails and feet.

The Body Shop (*www.bodyshop.com*)
Good value skin and hair care with an environmentally friendly approach.

Borghese (*www.borghese.com*)
Luxury skin and bodycare, enriched by the spa waters of Montecatini in Italy.

BriteSmile (*www.britesmile.com*)
The world's leading dental bleaching system, which uses a light-activated gel to lighten teeth by up to eleven shades in less than one hour.

Central London School of Reflexology
Maiden Lane, Covent Garden, London WC2E 7JS.
Telephone +44 (0)7240 1438

Christian Dior (*www.dior.com*)
Prestige French beauty brand renowned for fabulous fragrances, inspired make-up and hi-tech skincare.

Clarins (*www.clarins.com*)
Leading French skincare producers based on plant extracts and also famous for their secret but super-effective massage technique.

Clinique (*www.clinique.com*)
Great body and haircare sits alongside serious skincare. Particularly good for those with problem complexions.

Crabtree & Evelyn (*www.crabtree-evelyn.com*)
English-style luxuries for the home, from the kitchen to the bathroom and even the garden.

Decleor (*www.decleor.com*)
Intensive skin and bodycare based on the potency of active essential oils for wellbeing and harmony.

Elemis (*www.elemis.com*)
Esteemed aromatherapy skincare, bath and body lines, favoured by leading spas around the world.

Elizabeth Arden (*www.elizabetharden.com*)
Pioneering anti-ageing skincare, plus colour combined with treatment and well-loved fragrances.

ESPA (*www.espaonline.com*)
Wonderful essential-oil-based products for bath, body, skin and home, plus fantastic treatments in world-leading spas.

Estée Lauder (*www.esteelauder.com*)
Famed for the advanced technology and groundbreaking research that brings consumers smarter beauty with state of the art formulae.

Guerlain (*www.guerlain.com*)
One of the world's greatest perfume houses. Steeped in family heritage that now extends to make-up, skincare and a fêted bronzing range.

Keet Clinic
Leading UK podiatry clinic that also offers on-site physiotherapy, reflexology and homeopathy.
29 Maiden Lane, Covent Garden, London WC2E 7JS.
Telephone +44 (0)20 7240 1438

Kiehl's Since 1851 (*www.kiehls.com*)
Apothecary-style range from New York that's become a cult beauty brand with best-selling hair and skincare for men and women.

Lancôme (*www.lancome.com*)
Trend-setting make-up collections alongside great skincare and classic modern fragrances.

Martyn Maxey
18 Grosvenor Street, London W1
+44 (0)20 7629 6161
Leading Mayfair hair and beauty salon.

Molton Brown (*www.moltonbrown.com*)
Slick British brand aimed at mixing wellbeing and lifestyle in modern products for top to toe care.

Origins (*www.origins.com*)
Funky aromatherapy-inspired range for balancing mind and body. Offers a complete range of beauty and home products.

Orla Kiely (*www.orlakiely.com*)
Known for her distinct patterns and contemporary designs, Orla Kiely now produces a full line of accessories and clothing.

Shu Uemura (*www.shu-uemura.co.jp*)
The original make-up artist's own brand. Includes a stunning palette of colour for the face and state of the art skincare with a natural twist.

Spa Resorts

Chiva Som (*www.chivasom.com*)
Chiva Som Hua Hin
73/4 Petchkasem Road, Hua Hin,
Prachuab Khirikham 77110,
Thailand.
Tel : +66 (0) 3253 6536
Fax : +66 (0) 3251 1154
e-mail: reservation@chivasom.com

Hotel Fortina (*www.hotelfortina.com*)
Tigné Seafront, Sliema SLM 15, Malta
Telephone: +356 (0)213 42976, (+356) 2134 3380,
Fax: +356 (0)21339388
e-mail: info@hotelfortina.com

Space NK (*www.spacenk.com*)
Cool beauty boutique featuring an eclectic mix of brands from around the world. Complemented by an expanding eponymous line of tools, hair and bodycare and fragrance.

Vaishaly Patel (*www.vaishaly.com*)
51 Paddington Steet, London N1
+44 (0) 20 8907 5617
Celebrity facialist, famed for her lymphatic drainage technique, as well as her skill in threading for elegant eyebrows.

Yves Saint Laurent (*www.ysl.com*)
Designer fragrance and luxury skincare that successfully combines performance and aesthetics.

Clothes and accessories: Models' own.
Bags: Orla Kiely.
Homeware: Models' own and a selection from House of Fraser, Oxford Street, London (*www.houseoffraser.com*)

The New Facercise: Give Yourself a Natural Facelift
Carole Maggio, Pan Books
0330 49015 X

Further Information

For details of your nearest Body Control Pilates teacher, plus a wide range of Pilates equipment, books, videos and accessories, send a stamped addressed envelope to:

The Body Control Pilates Association
PO Box 29061
London WC2H 9TB
England
+44 (0) 20 7379 3734

Or visit the Body Control Pilates website at
www.bodycontrol.co.uk

A capsule collection of comfortable, hi-performance sportswear is available to buy on the internet www.bodycontrolclothing.com or via mail order on +44 (0)1858 469 588

Other Body Control Pilates books

BODY CONTROL THE PILATES WAY
0 330 36945 8 / £7.99

THE MIND–BODY WORKOUT
0 330 36946 6 / £12.99

PILATES THE WAY FORWARD
0 330 37081 2 / £12.99

PILATES THROUGH THE DAY:
The Morning Energizer / 0 330 37327 7 / £2.99
The Desk Reviver / 0 330 37328 5 / £2.99
The Evening Relaxer / 0 330 37329 3 / £2.99
Off to Sleep / 0 330 37330 7 / £2.99

THE OFFICIAL BODY CONTROL PILATES MANUAL
0 330 39327 8 / £12.99

PILATES GYM
0 330 48309 9 / £12.99

THE BODY CONTROL PILATES BACK BOOK
0 330 48311 0 / £9.99

THE BODY CONTROL PILATES
POCKET TRAVELLER
0 330 49106 7 / £4.99

INTELLIGENT EXERCISE WITH PILATES & YOGA
0 333 98952 X / £16.99

These are available from all good bookshops,
or can be ordered direct from:
Book Services By Post
PO Box 29
Douglas
Isle of Man IM99 IBQ

Credit card hotline +44 (0) 1624 675 137
Postage and packing free in the UK

Watch out for new titles!